Goodbye ARFID, Hello Food!

Fast & Effective 3-Step Process That Helps Reduce & Eliminate Food Phobia

Glenn Robertson

First published by Ultimate World Publishing 2025
Copyright © 2025 Glenn Robertson

ISBN

Paperback: 978-1-923425-59-0
Ebook: 978-1-923425-60-6

Glenn Robertson has asserted his rights under the Copyright, Designs and Patents Act 1988 to be identified as the author of this work. The information in this book is based on the author's experiences and opinions. The publisher specifically disclaims responsibility for any adverse consequences which may result from use of the information contained herein. Permission to use information has been sought by the author. Any breaches will be rectified in further editions of the book.

All rights reserved. No part of this publication may be reproduced, stored in or introduced into a retrieval system, or transmitted in any form, or by any means (electronic, mechanical, photocopying, recording or otherwise) without the prior written permission of the author. Any person who does any unauthorised act in relation to this publication may be liable to criminal prosecution and civil claims for damages. Enquiries should be made through the publisher.

Cover design: Ultimate World Publishing
Layout and typesetting: Ultimate World Publishing
Editor: Marinda Wilkinson
Cover Image Copyright: March Studio-Shutterstock.com

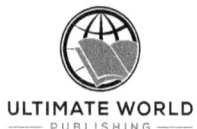

Ultimate World Publishing
Diamond Creek,
Victoria Australia 3089
www.writeabook.com.au

Disclaimer

This book is intended to provide general information and support for individuals dealing with Avoidant Restrictive Food Intake Disorder (ARFID) and those looking to understand it better. While the advice and strategies shared here are based on the author's experience in providing ARFID therapy, it is important to note that each person's journey with ARFID is unique.

This book is not a substitute for professional medical, psychological or nutritional advice. If you or someone you care about is experiencing severe symptoms or challenges related to ARFID, it is strongly recommended to seek personal guidance from a licensed healthcare provider, therapist or nutritionist who specialises in eating disorders.

The techniques and suggestions in this book are meant to be supportive tools, but they should not replace individualised care. Always consult with your healthcare team before making any significant changes to your eating habits or treatment plan.

Taking care of your physical and mental health is a priority, and this book aims to offer insight, hope and strategies for managing ARFID. Your wellbeing is a journey, and with the right support, you can make progress towards healing and growth.

Contents

Disclaimer iii
Introduction 1
How this book can help 3
How to get the most out of this book 5
Set your expectations 9

Chapter 1: ARFID INFORMATION: In Plain English 13
    What is ARFID? 14
    Types of ARFID 15
    Signs of ARFID 20
    What causes ARFID? 22
    ARFID onset in late childhood and beyond ... 24
    Emetophobia 26
    Chapter summary and key points 28

Chapter 2: STEP ONE: Understand How Your Mind Works 29
    This is what you will learn in Step One 30
    Learning to unlearn 31

Conscious vs. subconscious mind	32
Understanding what a 'part' of the mind means	35
What is a scientific eater?	36
Identifying the food fears holding you back	37
The power of perception	39
Your food instinct – the gatekeeper	41
List your BEST reasons for change	44
What is your learning style?	47
Information + emotion = change	49
Chapter summary and key points	50

Chapter 3: STEP TWO: Talk to Your Subconscious Mind — 51

This is what you will learn in Step Two	52
Your story (how did you get here?)	53
How to talk to your food instinct (your gatekeeper)	58
Choose your future – the left or right path?	67
Chapter summary and key points	76

Chapter 4: STEP THREE: Choose to be the Boss of Your Mind — 77

This is what you will learn in Step Three	78
Feel the power of your mind – the pendulum	79
Choice – the only thing you really own	84
It's time to be the leader of your mind	85
What is acceptable for a scientific eater?	87
Anticipatory anxiety (phobia vs. normal nerves)	90
Take the trainer wheels off your bicycle!	91
Time to be a food explorer!	93
What does the recovery path look like?	95
Chapter summary and key points	98

Contents

Chapter 5: BONUS SECTION: Keeping You Strong	**99**
Extra insights you'll learn in this bonus section	100
Building trust	101
Rating food	102
Plank of wood story – your 'safety net' around food	105
Manager's sandwich strategy	111
Motivation ideas	116
Guidance for parents	118
Chapter summary and key points	123
Cheat sheet for ARFID therapy success	124
Hypnosis: uses in ARFID therapy	127
Afterword	**131**
Acknowledgements	**133**
About The Author	**135**
Glenn as a Speaker	**137**
ARFID Therapy, Products, Resources and Assistance	**139**
Special offer – free ARFID roadmap	140
Free video – What is ARFID?	141
ARFID Food Phobia Therapy with Glenn Robertson	142
Complimentary 15-minute Zoom discovery call appointment	144
ARFID Australia support group	145
ARFID therapy online options	147
Appendix A	**151**
Appendix B	**153**
Testimonials	**159**

Introduction

If you are reading these words, it means that you (or someone you know and love) has ARFID.

Avoidant Restrictive Food Intake Disorder (ARFID) is a recognised eating disorder. It is not fussy or picky eating. It's more serious than that.

This book is for parents of an ARFID child, carers of people with ARFID, and most importantly, it is for anyone living with ARFID.

The **3-step ARFID therapy process** outlined in these pages will show you how the ARFID mind CAN change.

My goal is that everyone who reads this book will have the knowledge to help themselves (or their ARFID loved one) to be able to eat and explore new food without the old feelings of fear and disinterest holding them back.

Over the past 10 years I have worked with over 2,500 children, teenage and adult ARFID eating disorder clients.

> **The vast majority of my clients reduce or eliminate their ARFID food phobia during their first 90-minute therapy session.**

They do this by following the simple 3-step process outlined in this book.

I will guide you through these 3 simple steps as if you are sitting in my clinic having your own personal ARFID Food Phobia Therapy session.

The 3-step process is so simple that children as young as 8 can grasp the concepts. Nearly 75% of my ARFID clients are aged between 8 and 18.

I often use hypnosis in my therapy sessions, however the 3-step process outlined in this book helps most clients to release their ARFID behaviours even without the use of hypnosis.

This book gives you the knowledge and tools to say **Goodbye ARFID, Hello Food!**

Glenn Robertson

ARFID Specialist, Hypnotist, Psychotherapist

www.ARFIDtherapy.com

How this book can help

Regardless of the reason (or reasons) you have ARFID, this book can help you to better understand your mind and give you the tools to reduce or eliminate your ARFID feelings and behaviours.

There are many pathways that may contribute to a person developing ARFID:

- Physical (food) trauma

- Emotional trauma

- Sensory processing challenges

- Heightened anxiety (GAD)

- ADHD, autism, PDA, hypermobility

- Interoceptive awareness challenges

- Personality traits.

The information in this book cuts the cord that binds the initial ARFID inducing event (or events) with the ongoing and strong anxiety created by that event (or events).

How to get the most out of this book

This is a short instructional book based on thousands of clinical hours of working with ARFID clients.

I have distilled the ARFID Food Phobia Therapy process down to its most succinct and helpful form.

The 3-step process is designed to help your inner mind to change the way it feels and reacts around food.

> **ARFID therapy 3-step process**
>
> **1. Understand** how your mind works
>
> **2. Talk** to your subconscious mind
>
> **3. Decide** to be the boss of your mind

If you are a parent of a child (aged 8+) with ARFID, I suggest you read the book completely through first by yourself. Then you can read (or summarise) the book together with your child and do the short activities contained in each of the 3-step process chapters.

For adults and teenagers with ARFID, I encourage you to do the activities as you read each chapter of the book.

This book is designed to give you the same experience and outcome as if you were attending a face-to-face ARFID therapy session with me personally.

> **It is an immersive experience. As you read, your mind will be challenged about what it thinks, and how it thinks.**
>
> **Reading the book with an open mind IS THE THERAPY.**

Although you may read the book through quickly the first time, you may want to go back and re-read parts that resonate with you.

The stories and metaphors in this book will speak to a deeper part of your mind. Some stories you will connect with more than others. That's okay. This book is a catch-all for many different types of ARFID, so it's natural to connect with parts that speak directly to your lived experience.

Your job is just to enjoy the book and let your mind make the internal connections and changes in its own way.

The best attitude to hold while reading this book is one of curiosity and positive expectancy.

How to get the most out of this book

Thousands of people before you have experienced a positive outcome from following this 3-step process.

Now it's your turn.

Set your expectations

When someone attends an appointment with me in my clinic, they expect to experience change. By reading this book and following the simple 3-step process, you can also expect to experience some change.

> **A change in your thinking. A change in your understanding. And most importantly, a change in your behaviour and feelings around food.**

Change can be small, medium or large. And change is an ongoing process.

After reading and absorbing the concepts in this book, you may find that you begin to feel differently around food.

- Maybe you won't notice food as much. Food is around you but doesn't trigger you like it once did.

- Maybe you'll notice that you can easily reach out and explore food without the old feelings holding you back.

- Maybe your old overwhelming gag feeling around new food just isn't as strong, or has completely disappeared.

When I ask my clients how they feel at the end of their ARFID therapy session, they often say they feel just the same. They don't feel as if anything has changed … until they try some new food.

And then they notice the old negative feelings have reduced or disappeared.

So I invite you to hold an attitude of curiosity and positive expectancy. Read the book, enjoy the stories. See yourself in the stories and make them your own.

Your subconscious mind learns through story, creativity, imagination, emotion and belief.

> **If you read with a sense of curiosity and an open mind, you have every chance of letting go of your old food feelings, and experiencing the food freedom you have been looking for.**

Oh, and by the way, this journey can sometimes be emotional. Often when we do something important in our lives, we get emotional. That's natural.

Most clients who undertake this ARFID therapy 3-step process are sceptical at the beginning. They can't understand how listening to stories can reduce their negative feelings and emotions around food.

But for most of my clients, change happens. And it usually happens during their first 90-minute therapy session, by following the 3-step process.

This book is designed to give you the experience of an ARFID therapy session, taking you through the 3-step process at your own pace. Here's an overview of what we'll cover:

Set your expectations

- **ARFID Information: In plain English**

This will give you important information about ARFID to get you ready for the 3-step process.

- **STEP ONE: Understand how your mind works**

This is where I give you a tour of your mind. This will demystify how your mind works and show you WHY the mind makes ARFID thoughts and feelings.

- **STEP TWO: Talk to your subconscious mind**

This is where I show you HOW you can talk to your mind. We get up close and personal with the part of your mind that is giving you the ARFID thoughts and feelings.

- **STEP THREE: Choose to be the boss of your mind**

This is where the rubber hits the road. When you truly understand something, the fear is diminished, and you can start to make decisions without outdated and unhelpful emotions holding you back. This is where **you become the BOSS** and decide to reach out and explore new food.

Your journey with the ARFID therapy 3-step process begins right now. Enjoy!

Chapter 1

ARFID INFORMATION:
In Plain English

'You are never too young to learn, never too old to change.'

Russell M Nelson

'Knowledge will make you free.'

Socrates

What is ARFID?

ARFID is the acronym for **Avoidant Restrictive Food Intake Disorder**.

ARFID is a recognised eating disorder, as serious as anorexia and bulimia, and is listed in the *DSM-5* (*The Diagnostic and Statistical Manual of Mental Disorders*).

> **ARFID is a condition that causes the person to limit the amount and type of food they eat.**

A person with ARFID will avoid and restrict food, however this is NOT due to any negative body image or a desire to lose weight.

ARFID is usually the result of:

- A past trauma around food and/or eating
- A heightened sensory sensitivity to the smell, sight, touch or taste of food
- A lack of interest in food or eating (sometimes accentuated by autism, ADHD, hypermobility, general anxiety disorder, interoceptive challenges, etc.)
- Or a combination of the above.

ARFID is NOT fussy or picky eating. Whereas fussy eating is usually a phase that a child will grow out of, ARFID behaviour generally starts in early childhood and can last a lifetime if left untreated.

The ARFID person usually has a very small list of 'safe foods' that limits their nutritional intake. This can lead to long-term detrimental health problems.

Often the ARFID diet is called a 'toddler' or 'beige' diet, as most foods are refined carbohydrates and high in unhealthy fats and sugars. A typical ARFID diet might include white bread, biscuits, chicken nuggets, chips and sweets, with very limited fresh fruit, vegetables or protein.

> **For the ARFID person, their 'non safe' foods can produce negative emotional and/or physical reactions.**

If an ARFID person is forced or persuaded to try one of their 'non-safe' foods, it usually results in heightened anxiety, stress, tantrums, tears, gagging, vomiting or shutdown and avoidance.

The NIH (National Institutes of Health, USA) estimate that ARFID effects up to 4% of the population.

It is important to remember that ARFID sufferers are not doing this behaviour deliberately or consciously.

Types of ARFID

Someone with ARFID has a small list of 'safe' foods and may show indifference towards eating food.

Food may make them anxious and nervous. They might have heightened negative emotional reactions when they feel pressured to eat 'new' foods. Or food may have become of such low interest that it is easy for them to forget to eat.

Someone with ARFID is not deliberately creating issues for themselves with food. These strong food 'feelings' bubble up from deep inside, independent of conscious logical thought.

There are four main types (or categories) of ARFID:

Avoidant
SENSORY-BASED ARFID

Characterised by strong aversions to certain food textures, tastes, colours or smells, leading to a limited diet due to sensory sensitivities.

Aversive
FEAR-BASED ARFID

Significant fear of negative consequences associated with eating, such as choking, vomiting or experiencing gastrointestinal discomfort. This fear can lead to avoidance of certain foods or food groups.

Restrictive
LACK OF INTEREST

Characterised by a general disinterest or lack of motivation towards eating, potentially leading to insufficient food intake and nutritional deficiencies.

ARFID Plus
COMBINATION OF ISSUES

Where ARFID is a combination of two or more types, or is combined with other factors such as autism, ADHD, anxiety (GAD), OCD, hypermobility and interoceptive challenges.

Avoidant ARFID

This is where certain foods are avoided because of their sensory characteristics.

People with this type of ARFID may have a form of sensory processing disorder (or heightened sensory awareness), where they feel overwhelmed and disgusted by the texture, smell and appearance of certain foods.

For example, if the person hates mushy textures, then any foods perceived as being mushy create a heightened stress (avoidant) response.

As the years go on, anxiety and fear build on each other. Often the base textural/sensory experience can diminish over time (naturally or with therapy), but it is the underlying fear that the mind has built up around the food experience (e.g. mushy) that is the barrier to change.

Aversive ARFID

This is driven by a fear of negative consequences.

Imagine if you got food poisoning by eating a certain food from a certain shop. You would be reluctant to return to the shop and buy that food item in the future.

Now imagine that fear magnified and the feeling spread across many foods.

People with aversive ARFID may have had an experience (or just be afraid) of choking, vomiting, an allergic reaction, nausea, constipation, etc. Often this experience happened in the past, and there is no current risk of it reoccurring.

This drive to avoid a negative food experience can turn into an extreme fear (or phobia) and can severely restrict the type and quantity of foods eaten, and eventually lead to nutritional deficiencies.

Restrictive ARFID

This group has a low interest in food and just don't feel motivated to eat. Eating feels like a chore and they stick to a narrow range of foods because they don't get any pleasure from eating. And because of this, they have no incentive to expand their food range.

For some people with ADHD, eating is low priority. When they are focused on something that interests them, they often forget to eat. Or there may be a disconnect with interoceptive cues like hunger and appetite regulation.

Adult ARFID

This is where ARFID behaviours have persisted into the adult years. Social, work, relationship and family dynamics place extra pressure on adults where food is constantly a challenge.

Being a role model for children, attending work functions, attending parties and celebrations, holidaying with friends – all of these should be pleasurable, but for the ARFID adult they are daunting.

Often ARFID in adults is a continuation of a childhood disorder. However change IS possible at any age.

ARFID Plus

This is where ARFID seems to be a combination of two or more types, or is combined with other factors such as autism, ADHD, anxiety (GAD), OCD, hypermobility and interoceptive challenges.

NEDC (National Eating Disorders Collaboration, Australia) estimate that 21% of autistic people experience ARFID at some time in their life. Autism can generate stronger sensory responses to food that may also include altered hunger cues and uncomfortable feelings in the gut. Food is also unpredictable (seasonal, blemishes, differences across brands, etc.), and this can be an impediment to exploring new foods.

NEDC also estimate that up to 26% of people diagnosed with ARFID will also have ADHD, where distraction can easily lead to disinterest.

And the National Alliance for Eating Disorders USA estimate that over 75% of people presenting with ARFID have GAD (generalised anxiety). Anxiety is the fuel that sustains most ARFID behaviour.

Also, hypermobility not only effects the joint connective tissue, but can also affect the motility of the bowel resulting in prolonged gut discomfort, constipation, irritability, etc. This can lead to food aversion over time.

Summary

The different types of ARFID often overlap. An autistic person may also have underlying food trauma or heightened sensory awareness.

And someone who has experienced food trauma may also have a sensitive or nervous disposition.

> **After working with over 2,500 ARFID clients (of all types) I have found that reducing the mind's internal automatic anxious reaction to food can help reduce and even eliminate ARFID, regardless of the type of ARFID.**

The 3-step process outlined in this book is predominately focused on understanding and reducing this internal anxiety around food.

This means that even if there are comorbid challenges such as autism, ADHD, SPD, hypermobility, etc., there is still a realistic opportunity that the person can begin to explore 'new' foods without their old reactions holding them back.

And importantly, the 3-step process is complementary to any other therapy the ARFID person may be exploring.

Many parents and ARFID clients have reported that after undertaking the therapy outlined in this book, they have noticed increased benefits when seeing their dietician, occupational therapist, psychologist, etc.

Reducing the internal anxiety and negative food feelings often opens the door for people to be able to engage more fully in complementary therapies.

Signs of ARFID

There are certain signs that will give an indication if someone is exhibiting ARFID behaviour. The signs can vary across the various ARFID types.

ARFID INFORMATION: In Plain English

The following list includes some of the most common signs that someone may be struggling with ARFID:

- Small list of safe foods

- Inability to 'try' new foods

- Gagging or vomiting when pushed to eat new foods

- Lots of food rules (specific brands and packaging, foods touching on plate, etc.)

- Prolonged disinterest in eating food (low hunger signals)

- Health deteriorating due to restrictive food intake

- Oversensitivity to food smells, tastes and textures

- Actively avoiding social situations that involve food

- Unpredictable behaviour around food

- Difficulty eating meals with family or friends

- Eating very slowly

- Food jagging (sudden refusal to eat foods they ate previously)

- Tantrums or excessive negative emotions when presented with 'new' food

- Difficulty transitioning from liquid to mushy to solid foods

- Take own food on vacations, camps, etc.

- Food choices are typically bland (beige, toddler diet).

Someone with ARFID may have one or more of the above behaviours or reactions to food.

ARFID can be confirmed by consulting an eating disorder specialist or relevant medical practitioner.

However, regardless of whether a formal diagnosis of ARFID has been obtained, the ARFID therapy process outlined in this book will assist the ARFID person to understand and reduce their unwanted feelings around food.

What causes ARFID?

ARFID is not a one-size-fits-all diagnosis. There can be many different causes of ARFID. One of the most common causes is where ARFID is triggered by a childhood mini trauma.

To the outside person, the trauma may appear insignificant. But to the ARFID person, their mind and body experiences the trauma as a major negative emotional event.

The following table contains a list of the common childhood mini traumas that can create ARFID behaviour:

Reflux	Transition to solid foods
Colic	Constipation
Food allergies	Gastro
Tongue & lip tie	Choking
Tonsilitis	Vomiting

Vaccination reaction	Hospital/operation
Reaction to medication	Undiagnosed coeliac
Moving home/school/country	Attending creche/childcare

Sometimes ARFID behaviour is observable from birth. But for others, they may have been eating quite normally until one of the above events occurred when they were a baby or toddler (or even later as a teen or adult).

It's as if a part of the mind associates food with the feeling of discomfort and pain, and develops an overwhelming mistrust of food.

Some individual or personality traits can also contribute towards ARFID, including those listed in the following table:

Autism	ADHD
Hypermobility	Sensory processing disorder
Teen or adult food trauma	GAD (general anxiety disorder)
Oversensitive nature	Separation anxiety
Interoceptive awareness imbalance	PDA (pathological demand avoidance) and ODD

In my practice I have found that regardless of how and when the ARFID behaviour started, the fuel that keeps the internal food fear and disinterest burning is ANXIETY.

It's as if the person grows up, but a part of their mind continues to experience the pain, discomfort and mistrust around food with the same emotional reactivity and intensity as a small child. A part of the mind continues to behave the same way it did when the trauma occurred all those years ago.

The chart that follows will give you a pictorial look at what pushes someone over the 'ARFID line'. The ARFID line is where the internal, subconscious, uncomfortable feelings around food push into conscious awareness. ARFID behaviour is often a combination of a number of factors.

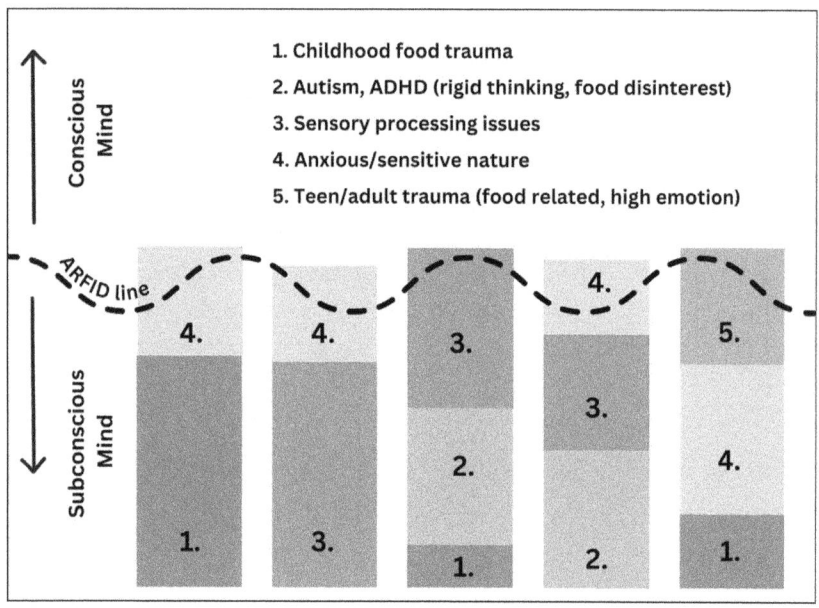

ARFID onset in late childhood and beyond

Isolated mini trauma

ARFID generally presents in the formative years between birth and 4 years of age. However sometimes ARFID behaviour may seem to start later on, in the primary school or teenage years (or even later).

In my experience, this later onset is primarily due to something triggering a person who is predisposed to ARFID.

For example, a person may have a highly anxious nature and yet appears to be eating normally up until 8 years of age.

Then they go to a party and choke on a piece of fruit or candy. Or they have a nasty bout of gastro. They may even require assistance from a doctor or hospital. But the experience has been traumatic (to them).

Due to the pre-existing underlying heightened anxiety condition, the food trauma receives heightened attention and emotion from the mind, and food and anxiety become firmly linked together.

From that moment forward, food becomes something the mind mistrusts, as it has the potential to cause a similar trauma.

This trauma is locked in at a subconscious level.

The conscious mind may be able to think about the trauma situation rationally and realise that food is not at fault, but the subconscious mind believes that if food can do this once, it can do it again. And so the subconscious mind becomes overprotective around food.

Some other common 'late onset' ARFID trigger events include gastroparesis, gut motility issues, emotional trauma, severe reaction to an emergency medical event, gastroenteritis, and even just witnessing a trauma associated with food (e.g. a choking incident).

When I'm anxious I eat less

When someone is anxious, the fight/flight/freeze mechanism is triggered in the subconscious mind and the body gets ready to deal with a perceived threat.

When the body is in protection mode, it switches off the desire for food and rest.

Fear triggers the sympathetic nervous system (fight/flight response), whereas eating and digestion occur in the parasympathetic nervous system (rest/digest).

You cannot be in both systems at the same time.

When food has given someone a heightened feeling of fear, the body moves into the sympathetic nervous system.

For some people, this subconscious food/fear/discomfort link has become so strong, that anytime they feel nervous, stressed or upset, their subconscious mind keeps food away as the first line of defence in dealing with the feeling.

Emetophobia

Emetophobia is a fear of vomiting. Maybe the person experienced a trauma (e.g. choking incident) around food and vomited, and this resulted in their mind creating an extreme aversion to the experience.

Or maybe the person just saw someone else sick or unwell.

Someone with emetophobia often feels unwell when they hear someone even say the word 'vomit', or see a picture or movie where someone is unwell.

They may also be overly focused on checking expiry dates on foods, be cautious about food preparation safety and hygiene standards. Excessive washing of hands is also common.

They may refuse to eat leftovers in the fridge or food that is not 'fresh'.

Someone with ARFID may feel nauseous or even gag around new food, but the person with emetophobia has an extreme fear of vomiting that expands beyond the interaction with food.

ARFID and emetophobia are not the same

Emetophobia is usually the result of a trauma experienced by someone who is predisposed to heightened levels of anxiety and stress.

In my experience, emetophobia is usually more difficult to shift than ARFID, however emetophobia often responds positively to the therapy strategy outlined in this book.

Chapter summary and key points

- ARFID is where a person has a small number of safe foods, and has a **negative emotional or physical reaction** when pushed to eat outside of their safe group of foods.

- Someone with ARFID may **want to eat, but they just can't**. It's as if their mind and body won't let them try the new food.

- The link between **autism, ADHD, anxiety** and ARFID is strong.

- There are 4 main types of ARFID, but the fuel that keeps ARFID burning over the years is the **subconscious feeling of ANXIETY** around food.

  Now that you have a clearer understanding of ARFID, you are ready to explore the 3-step process that I use with all of my ARFID clients.

  Of course, if you were attending a personal ARFID therapy session in my clinic, I would tailor the therapy to your specific personality type and reference the specific events in your life history that are relevant to ARFID.

  But regardless of your individual ARFID type, the following pages will give you (or your child) an opportunity to experience in your own home, the ARFID therapy process that I have used with over 2,500 clients.

  Okay, let's turn the page and begin!

Chapter 2

STEP ONE:

Understand How Your Mind Works

'If you change the way you look at things, the things you look at change.'

Wayne Dyer

'Until you make the unconscious conscious, it will direct your life and you will call it fate.'

Carl Jung

This is what you will learn in Step One

- ✓ You have more than one **mind**, and they work in very different ways.

- ✓ Changing your **perception** can change how you **feel** around food.

- ✓ Becoming a **scientific eater** will change how you **think** about food.

- ✓ Why your **food instinct** is the **gatekeeper** of all of your interactions with food.

- ✓ Where the **ARFID thoughts** live in your mind.

STEP ONE is all about understanding how your **MIND** works.

Your feelings around food have been created for a very good reason.

Once you are clear on the reason, you'll be able to help your mind to think differently.

I'm here to guide you, so let's get started!

STEP ONE: Understand How Your Mind Works

Learning to unlearn

The majority of ARFID behaviours are learned responses to past negative events.

The good news is that if something can be learned, it can also be unlearned. You can learn to do it differently. Most people are capable of change, even if it's small.

In the next three chapters, I am going to show you how to unlearn your ARFID and do it differently.

Humans are survivors. We have a built-in ability to remember when something is unpleasant so that we can avoid it in the future.

If an event is particularly unpleasant and a negative emotional reaction occurs, then a strong warning memory is created to make sure we do not repeat that activity or event again.

When we are young, these strong warning memories are created automatically (subconsciously), because we don't have life experience to know any different.

If a person can't swim, they go to a swimming coach who shows them the correct swimming technique, so they build confidence and stop being afraid of water. A coach can help us let go of old habits, so new and better habits can be formed.

And so it is with ARFID. Your mind (in the past) has learned certain things about food that has made it cautious, wary and disinterested.

I want to help your mind unlearn its worries about food, and give you back the power to be in charge of your food decisions, rather than your mind swamping you with those old unnecessary negative feelings.

Remember, if you can learn something, you can also learn to do it differently.

Conscious vs. subconscious mind

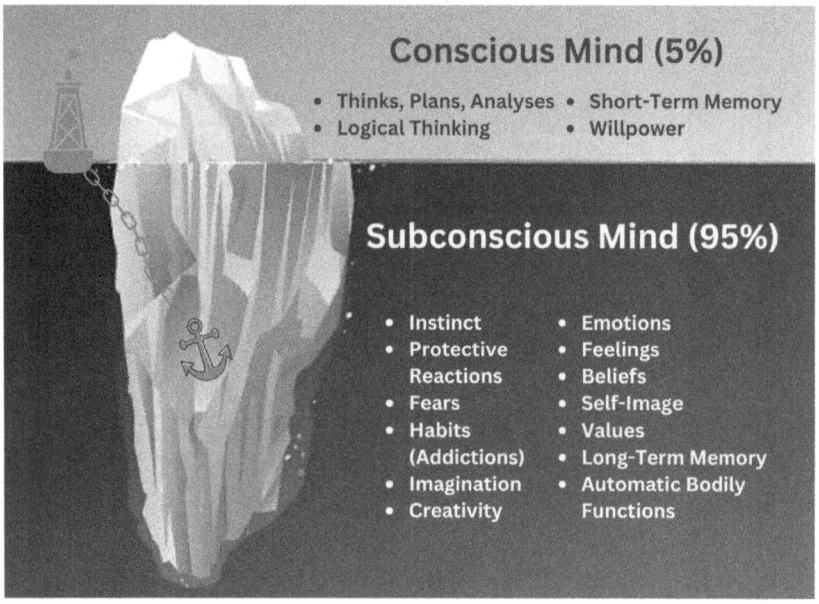

Whenever someone comes into my office for ARFID therapy, I always ask them, 'How many minds do you think you have?'

Most people say one. But in fact, we've got TWO distinct parts of our mind. ARFID lives in one part of the mind. When we finally understand which part that is, we can begin our journey to ARFID freedom.

> **Your two minds are the CONSCIOUS MIND and the SUBCONSCIOUS MIND.**

STEP ONE: Understand How Your Mind Works

When you look at the picture of the iceberg in this section, the conscious mind is that small part of the iceberg above the water line, and the subconscious mind is the larger part below.

Let's start with your **conscious mind**.

The conscious mind is the part that you're using right now. You're using your eyes to look at this page. Maybe there's some music in the background you can hear. You can feel the chair on your legs. The five senses bring information into the conscious mind.

And in the conscious mind is our rational, logical, reasoning mind. It's the mind that we take to work and school each day. And in this conscious part of the mind is your short-term memory and willpower.

As you can see in the picture, the conscious mind is the small part of the iceberg.

Underneath the waterline is the **subconscious mind**.

The word 'sub' means under (a submarine is underwater), so the subconscious is the part of the mind that is under our conscious awareness.

The subconscious is the biggest part of the mind. Down in the subconscious mind is our long-term memory. NOTHING IS FORGOTTEN down there.

Our automatic reactions and our protective instincts are in the subconscious mind. So are our firmly held beliefs, our habits, our addictions, our emotions and creativity.

And down in the subconscious mind is also the automatic functioning of the body. Right now, as you're reading these words, your toenails are growing, your eyes are blinking, and your lungs are breathing. You're not deciding to do these things with your conscious mind, they are happening subconsciously.

So imagine the buoy in the iceberg picture represents something you want to consciously change or move. To your conscious mind it just looks like a buoy floating on the surface of the water.

You can see it with the conscious mind, but when you consciously try and move it or push it, you can't. It's because you can't see the part underneath the water that is chained and anchored in the iceberg of the subconscious mind.

No matter how hard you try to move it consciously, it doesn't budge. It's because the thing that is holding it in place and keeping it from moving is the chain and anchor that attaches it to the subconscious mind.

And THAT is the reason you're reading this book.

For years you've been using your conscious mind to try and change the way you feel and react around food, but no matter how hard you try, you just can't change.

It's because the feeling that is holding you back is anchored in your subconscious mind. You can't see it on the surface, and you don't know why it's blocking you.

Today, by reading this book, you will finally understand why your subconscious mind is behaving that way around food.

You will understand why it is giving you those unhelpful feelings around food.

STEP ONE: Understand How Your Mind Works

So let's keep going and find out what those feelings are and why they are there.

Understanding what a 'part' of the mind means

Often you hear people refer to a '**part**' of their mind.

Maybe you've heard someone say, '*I had a day off work and a part of me wanted to go to the gym, but another part of me just wanted to sit on the couch and watch Netflix.*'

In my clinic, I see many people who want to give up smoking and other negative and addictive behaviours.

The smoking clients that come to see me stand at the door and say, '*Glenn, I'm here to give up smoking. I know it's bad for my lungs. I know it's bad for my heart. And I know it's bad for my wallet because it's costing me a fortune!*'

And then they ALWAYS say, '*But there's a part of me that just wants to smoke!*'

So smokers get it. They know there is a part of them that is focused on health and doing the right thing, and yet they're also aware of this other strong part that compels them to do the unwanted smoking behaviour.

That strong smoking part lives in the subconscious mind. It seems to be doing the opposite of what the conscious mind wants.

As you're reading these words, YOUR subconscious mind is also listening.

The part of your mind that is nervous, scared or reluctant to try new food, is listening.

This book speaks directly to THAT part of your mind.

And that part lives in the subconscious mind.

What is a scientific eater?

I want to help you become a **scientific eater**. Understanding what a scientific eater does, is a really important concept in this therapy process.

I think of a scientist as someone who does experiments.

So if I'm a scientific eater and I've got three foods in front of me that I've never tried before, I might say to myself, *'Glenn, you're a scientific eater. Just reach out, do an experiment and use your grown-up mind to decide if you like it or not, rather than letting another part of your mind decide automatically for you.'*

So I reach out for the first food and nervously pick it up, and as I try it my mind says, *'Whoa! That's pretty good.* **I like it**. *Where's that been all my life?'*

So I go for the second food and as I try it I think, *'It's okay. It's not my favourite, but I can eat it.'*

But when I try the third food item, as soon as it touches my tastebuds, I just don't like it. So I take it out and I put it on the plate and say, *'I'm not eating it. I don't like it.'*

A true scientist does an experiment and THEN makes up their mind based on the outcome. Not the other way around.

STEP ONE: Understand How Your Mind Works

So I'm going to help you become a scientific eater. And here's the good news: a scientific eater DOES NOT need to like everything that they try.

It is perfectly acceptable for a scientific eater to say, *'Yes, I like that'*, or *'No I don't like that'*. Your parents and friends don't like everything they try.

The 3-step process of letting go of ARFID has got nothing to do with you liking everything, but it has got everything to do with GIVING YOU BACK THE POWER to reach out and explore food without those old feelings shutting you down.

Identifying the food fears holding you back

So let's find out what those feelings, emotions or fears are that are holding you back from reaching out and exploring new food, or from even allowing you to think about trying new food.

> **One of the easiest ways of getting in touch with those feelings and emotions is by using our imagination.**

So I want you to use your imagination right now. Imagine that in front of you there is a plate, and on that plate is food that you don't currently eat.

You look at the food and think, *'Okay, I'm going to give this a try.'* But as your hand reaches out to pick up some of that food, and it starts to come towards your mouth, something inside of your mind says, *'Nooo, don't do it! Don't open your mouth.'* And you just can't do it.

If you were to describe THOSE feelings that stop you from putting that food in your mouth, (or if it does get into your mouth, the feelings that prevent you from swallowing it), what words would you use?

Some people say it's a feeling of fear. Others say they get this overwhelming feeling that they just don't want to do it. Some people say they are worried about the texture. Others think that it's 'gross'. And there are many other negative food feelings that people have shared with me over the years.

So right now, I'd like you to write down (in the space provided) what are the feelings and emotions that you experience as you imagine that new food coming towards your mouth.

They're just feelings. They don't need to make logical sense.

Some people say to me, *'I'm not quite sure, but it's as if there's an invisible wall in front of me, and even if I wanted to put that food into my mouth, well, I just can't. It's like my mind and body are just holding me back.'*

And other people say, *'Well, I'm just not interested. I just don't have the desire to reach out and try it, so I don't even think about it.'*

Others also say, *'It's only when somebody really insists, and forces me to try, then all of a sudden I start to feel those uncomfortable thoughts and feelings inside.'*

STEP ONE: Understand How Your Mind Works

Take a few moments and write down a few words about how trying new food, or thinking about new food, makes you FEEL:

_____

_____

_____

_____

_____

_____

_____

Good. These are the feelings that I will help you reduce as you work through this book.

The power of perception

Perception is really important because it impacts how we interact with the world. It affects every single area of our life.

So I want to tell you a story to help you get crystal clear on what perception really means, and how your PERCEPTION affects your FEELINGS around food.

Imagine you come to visit me in my clinic in Melbourne, Australia, and we decide to go out for a walk in the countryside. You're in the lead, and I'm following, and we're walking down a small dirt path.

As you're walking down this path you notice that there's long grass growing on either side of the path. It doesn't bother you.

As we keep walking you notice that the sun is getting low in the sky so the shadows are going across the path and it's getting darker. That doesn't bother you either. You keep walking.

And then you think to yourself, *'Hang on. I'm in Australia, the land of spiders and snakes!'* And in that very moment, out of the corner of your eye, you just notice something coiled up in the long grass next to the path.

If you're like me, this would be enough to make you panic. All of a sudden your hands get sweaty, your heart starts to pump quickly, and you get really nervous.

I'm behind you, and when I look over your shoulder I think I know what that thing looks like in the long grass, and I get really nervous as well.

But you're braver than me. So you gently go up to this thing in the grass, you shine your phone light on it, and then all of a sudden you turn around, say, *'Glenn, it's just an old garden hose.'* And we both start to relax and feel more comfortable.

STEP ONE: Understand How Your Mind Works

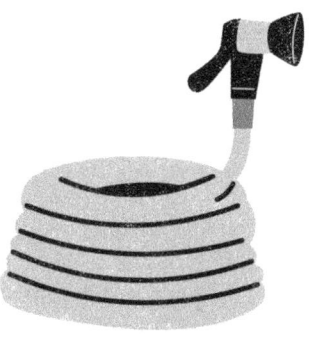 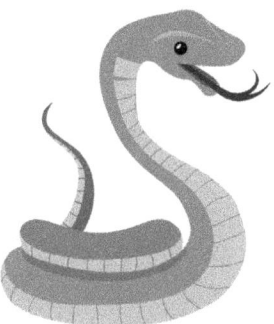

> **THAT'S PERCEPTION! Perception has got nothing to do with the thing. Perception is what our mind thinks the thing is.**

When our mind saw that shape in the grass, and it matched an image (or pattern) in our memory, our mind thought it was a snake. Our hands got sweaty, our heart started to beat, we had a physiological response, **because of a thought in our mind**. And yet it was never a snake.

So let's talk about your **food** perception.

I know for you, at some time in your past, your perception around food just got out of balance.

Through the 3-step process, I want to help bring your food perception back into balance.

Your food instinct – the gatekeeper

Our instinct is the part of the mind that is in charge of keeping us safe, to make sure that we survive.

Instinct resides in the limbic system within the subconscious mind. Any fearful and anxious memories formed around food are processed and stored in the amygdala (which is part of the limbic system).

When the amygdala responds to stress, it can disable the frontal lobes (conscious mind) and activate the fight/flight response.

The role of instinct is vitally important. It's the reason that you and I are here today. It's been working for thousands and millions of years to make sure that the human species survives.

> **The role of instinct is to keep us safe and to be aware of danger. To do this, instinct REMEMBERS and attaches EMOTION with the MEMORY.**

If something makes us uncomfortable, hurts us, injures us or is a dangerous situation, our instinct creates a memory pattern of that experience and stores it in the subconscious mind.

It also connects that pattern with the strong negative emotions created by that experience. These are the emotions created at the time and age you have the experience.

From that moment forward, instinct is always on the lookout to keep us safe from that pattern happening again.

> **The role of instinct is also to look for things that are PREDICTABLE and FAMILIAR. When things are the same, when things are predictable, instinct feels safe.**

If a young child is bitten by a dog and the fear, emotion or trauma is strong enough, the instinctive mind links heightened fear with dogs, and locks the experience in the subconscious memory.

Even though the child grows up, the subconscious fear often retains the same intensity. The intense toddler fear created around dogs when the incident occurred, is the same intense fear their mind gives them as a teen or an adult.

It's not mature fear. It's toddler fear felt in a mature body.

That's why the fear response may seem out of proportion. But it's just instinct doing its job. It's keeping us away from a pattern that had an intense negative emotional response in the past.

Instinct lives in the subconscious mind.

I want to help you with your instinct around food, because you're not doing these excessive food reactions deliberately. You have grown up. The intensity of those past instinctive reactions around food created by the younger you, are no longer relevant to the grown-up you that is here today.

I call this food instinct within your mind the gatekeeper.

The gatekeeper's role is to look out from the gate and let in things or people that it trusts, and to close the gate and keep out things that it doesn't trust.

If you like toast or plain biscuits, your gatekeeper may see those foods coming down the path and open up and quite happily let them in. But if toast arrives with something on it that you don't normally have, it will stay shut and won't let it in. It's as if the gatekeeper doesn't recognise it as food.

In the next chapter I want to talk with your gatekeeper (your food instinct).

> **YOU, the conscious mind, are not the one that is creating these negative feelings around food. These unwanted feelings are the automatic response from the food instinct within your subconscious mind.**

That's the part we're going to speak with.

List your BEST reasons for change

If we're going to do something new in life, or if we want to change an old pattern of behaviour, then we've got to have a really good reason for doing it.

I'd like you to use your imagination so we can find out your BEST reasons for change.

Imagine that in your mind there is a whiteboard filled with all of your food worries, your negative food memories, and your uncomfortable feelings around food. It's full of your disinterest in food. It's full of all of the embarrassing memories that involve food. Look how full that whiteboard appears. So many things!

Now imagine that I give you a magic eraser. And this magic eraser can wipe them all away.

So do that now. Imagine wiping that whiteboard in your mind right now and erasing all those old negative memories, feelings and thoughts around food. Scrub it clean. Good.

Now that you've done that, I want you to think about the activities, situations and life events that involve food, that you could now participate in and enjoy.

> **What would you be able to do, now that all that old food worry has been wiped out and gone?**

STEP ONE: Understand How Your Mind Works

I'd like you to write those things down in the space provided at the end of this section.

Some of my ARFID clients find this a difficult task, because they've been doing their old behaviour for so long.

So I'll list for you the most common responses that clients have shared with me over the years, and this may help you create your own list.

Parties and sleepovers: they want to be able to enjoy these times like their friends and not be worried about food.

School camps: normally impossible or stressful and embarrassing. They want to go to camp and not have to bring their own food or be in the 'special' line for food.

Vacation or holidays: usually they have to take along a bag of their safe food. They want to eat at different restaurants and have fun rather than only eating at restaurants that have hot chips and chicken nuggets.

School lunches: they would like some variety in their lunches and be able to choose something different from the canteen.

Sport: they want to be able to have an orange or food at half time, just like all of their teammates.

Takeout and cafes: as clients get older, they want to be able to hang out with friends at cafes or buy takeout without being the odd one out.

Partner: meeting a new partner and not being embarrassed about explaining food issues is a dream for many.

Work: being able to enjoy training or professional development days (where lunch is provided) would be great (rather than always panicking and missing out).

Family celebrations: birthdays, religious celebrations and family gatherings would be easier.

Dinner at home: knowing someone does not have to make a special meal for them would make dinnertimes more pleasant.

Restaurants: being able to go to a new restaurant without panicking would be great.

These are the reasons that people come to ARFID therapy.

They don't come to therapy to please a partner or to please a parent. They come to therapy for themselves, so they can enjoy life more. So they can start doing the things that they are currently missing out on, like the things in the above list.

After you've written down your reasons in the box provided, I want you to circle your top two reasons.

Once you've got your top two reasons, these will be your powerful motivators to help you get the most out of this ARFID therapy process.

STEP ONE: Understand How Your Mind Works

List how your life will change for the better, when the uncomfortable feelings around food become less and disappear.

1. _____

   _____

2. _____

   _____

3. _____

   _____

4. _____

   _____

5. _____

   _____

What is your learning style?

It's worth thinking about your learning style, because we all learn differently. Are you somebody that jumps in early and has a go, or do you hold back and process things cautiously? Are you perfectionistic, or rigid in your thinking? Are you a visual, auditory or kinesthetic learner?

Think about the things in your life that you learn easily. Maybe you're good at mathematics and logic and less adept at English and creativity – or maybe it's the other way around.

The ARFID therapy 3-step process will help you CHANGE your thinking and feeling around food.

Change just means learning to do something new. The way that you learn to do anything new in your life, is the way you will probably learn to do new food.

The beauty about learning something new is that we have permission to make mistakes. That's what learning is all about. Having a go, making mistakes and getting better.

It is also normal to feel nervous when we start learning something new.

Learning to do something new also tends to push us out of our comfort zone. When we are learning something new, we shouldn't expect to do it perfectly. If we don't get it quite right the first time, we learn, adjust and try again.

Learning is all about progress, not perfection. And so it is with food. Your mind will be absorbing a lot of information throughout this 3-step process, and at the right time you'll decide to do something new around food.

This is where understanding your learning style is important.

So don't compare yourself with anybody else. This is your race, your pace. And it doesn't matter if change is small, medium or large. All that matters is that you're learning, and heading in the right direction.

Information + emotion = change

The fastest way to experience change is to combine new information with emotion.

Information is assessed by the conscious mind.

Emotion is processed by the subconscious mind.

If the information we asses is accepted as true by the conscious mind, and if that information or experience triggers a strong positive emotion (belief, excitement, relief) in the subconscious mind, then change IS possible, and in most cases, inevitable.

Often, as I move through this 3-step process with clients, they cry or become emotional.

It's as if feelings that have been locked inside are finally released, because the person finally understands WHY they have been behaving that way around food.

There is a feeling of relief when they finally understand that they are not doing it consciously. They are doing it subconsciously.

Chapter summary and key points

- ✓ ARFID is a **subconscious problem,** not a conscious problem.

- ✓ It's okay to **feel nervous** and make mistakes when we attempt to learn something new.

- ✓ Your food instinct is only trying to **protect you**. It is not deliberately trying to make your life difficult around food.

- ✓ Your **perception can change** over time.

- ✓ A scientific eater is a food explorer. They decide if they like something **after they try** (not before).

Congratulations. You've completed the first step.

Instead of just having one way of thinking about ARFID and your mind, you can now look at things from a new perspective.

Your mind is now thinking differently.

Let's move on to Step Two and talk to your subconscious mind.

Chapter 3

STEP TWO:

Talk to Your Subconscious Mind

'People do not come into therapy to change their past, but their future.'

Milton Erickson

'The mind is like the stomach. It is not how much you put into it that counts, but how much it digests.'

Albert J Nock

This is what you will learn in Step Two

- ✓ A clearer **understanding** of your lifetime ARFID journey.

- ✓ How to **communicate** with your gatekeeper.

- ✓ You have the **power to choose** your future.

STEP TWO is all about **TALKING** to your subconscious mind.

It's about finding out why you developed ARFID feelings, and asking your mind to change.

And it's about getting clear on what you want, and making a decision about your future.

I'm here to support you every step of the way, so let's keep going!

STEP TWO: Talk to Your Subconscious Mind

Your story (how did you get here?)

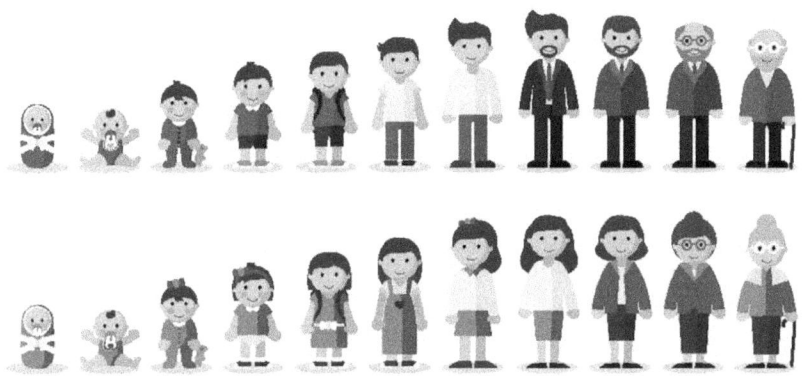

In the last two chapters you have learned some new information about ARFID and the mind.

> **Now it's time to take a look at YOUR STORY and why ARFID has been such a big part of your life.**

The story I'm about to tell you will be relevant to YOU, whether you are 8, 15, 27, 45, 60, 72 or any age in-between.

As you read this story, you might like to think about the parts that sound exactly like you.

So, let me tell you a story ...

Let's wind the clock all the way back to the first day that you were born.

And if that day was a normal birthing day, at some point you were probably placed in your mother's arms and your one-day-old-brain was probably thinking, *'This is pretty good. I feel loved, I feel warm, I feel protected, I feel safe. And when I'm hungry, somebody gives me something to eat.'*

But we now know more about that young you than anybody could see or know all those years ago.

- For some people, they arrive on the planet with heightened anxiety. That's their personality. As a young baby with anxiety, it means there is a natural tendency to be more cautious of anything new. It's as if the baby's system is always on high alert.

- Other people are born with an allergy, so that every time they eat something specific, they have a negative physical reaction to the food. And for that young body all those years ago, it's as if the instinct within their mind jumps up and says, *'What's going on? Why do we feel uncomfortable?'* At that young age, the mind doesn't know any better and food gets the blame most of the time.

- Some babies have extended periods of colic or reflux and have stomach pain. They may vomit regularly and feel unwell. Again, the baby's instinct just begins to join the dots and notes that whenever food is around they feel unwell. So a wariness develops around food.

- Maybe there was some gastro, a viral infection, acute constipation or medical emergency that required a hospital visit. If food is around and pain and discomfort is experienced, then to the young baby brain, food is the logical thing to blame.

- Maybe a simple choking incident created sufficient fear in that young mind, and food became the enemy.

- Some babies are comfortable taking milk, but when mushy and solid foods arrive, it feels different. That transition never really occurs. The cautious nature in the child pushes away the thing that makes them feel uncomfortable. And a cycle of fear and avoidance starts.

- Maybe that young child arrived with a neurodiverse brain (autism and/or ADHD). This may predispose some children to a natural cautiousness and a more rigid thinking process. Food is new and unpredictable, so the natural tendency is to stick to the things that are known. Known things are safer than unknown things.

- And sometimes food is just not as interesting as other things that are happening, so disinterest starts to develop.

- Maybe there were some interoceptive challenges. Maybe hunger signals, feeling full and feeling thirsty are not operating exactly how they should.

- Maybe that young child had increased sensory awareness. So the smell, texture and taste of some foods put them into sensory overload and they felt nervous and overwhelmed. So keeping food away was just like keeping bad feelings away.

So many maybes!

One (or a combination) of these things was most likely experienced by you (as the ARFID child) sometime in the first few years after birth.

And then maybe you went to kindergarten or childcare, and the teacher didn't know that you've already begun to have these really uncomfortable thoughts and feelings around food. And maybe the teacher said, *'Come on, sit there, eat the food like everybody else before you go and play.'*

But you can't do it, because there's just this feeling inside of your mind that won't let you feel comfortable around new food.

And even though your parents love you, I can guarantee they probably said this to you as you were growing up. *'Come on, you can do it. Look, I can eat the food, it's easy. There's nothing wrong with it. Just one mouthful. Come on, chew it, swallow it.'*

But you can't do it. Even if you want to please your parent, there's something inside of your mind and body that just won't let you do it. Dinnertimes were mostly stressful and food and anxiety grew stronger in your mind.

And then you go to school. Your good friends at school know that you don't eat everything, so they don't say anything, because that's what good friends do. But other people who don't know you so well, you might have heard them say, *'Come on, try it. We're eating it. Surely you can eat it. Is there a problem? Is there something wrong with you?'*

So not only are you nervous of food and you feel under pressure, but all of a sudden there's embarrassment that comes from peer pressure and the desire to fit in.

And in your teens and early 20s, the discomfort grows, because all of your friends are going to cafes and restaurants, but whenever you go you can't eat anything. You're the only one that is there eating chips or nothing at all.

Or you go to work and there's a training day. Lunch is provided and everybody else just goes and has whatever is provided, but you can't do it. And you feel as if you stand out.

Maybe you want to take that special person in your life out for dinner. But you can't do it. They want to go to an Indian,

STEP TWO: Talk to Your Subconscious Mind

Thai or Mexican restaurant, but you just can't go there unless you pre-inspect the menu to find out if there is anything you can eat.

And here you are today. It's as if something in your mind and body says, *'That's it. Food has given us too much trouble over all these years. We're going to eat our safe foods, because we trust them. They're safe and predictable. But we're not eating anything else. It's too difficult and too much pressure. It makes us feel bad. So we're not even going to think about doing new food.'*

And you feel that for your whole life food has restricted you from doing and enjoying what everyone else does so easily.

Does that sound like you?

Does that sound like the reason you're reading this book?

Yes?

Well, I understand.

And I know you are not doing it deliberately.

There is another part of your mind that is giving you these restrictive feelings around food.

That's the part this book is speaking to.

Let's talk directly to that ARFID part of your mind now.

How to talk to your food instinct (your gatekeeper)

You have now arrived at a very powerful and important part of the 3-step process.

So far you've learned that the **subconscious mind** and the **conscious mind** do different things.

You understand **perception.**

You are clear on the choices for a **scientific eater**.

And you know that your food instinct is like a **gatekeeper**. It (not YOU) decides how you feel and behave around food.

So now is the time to talk to your gatekeeper. This is the strong food instinct within your mind.

Your gatekeeper is the part of your mind that's been flooding you with all of those unnecessary thoughts and feelings around food.

Your gatekeeper is the part of your mind that's been holding you back for years from doing what you want to do around food.

Your gatekeeper lives in the subconscious mind.

Your gatekeeper normally doesn't speak or listen to your conscious mind, but there is a way.

We need to bring the gatekeeper out of your mind so we can talk with it.

The best way to do this is by using your powerful imagination.

STEP TWO: Talk to Your Subconscious Mind

So right now, stretch out your arm in front of you, palm facing upwards. You can let your arm rest on the table or your lap for comfort.

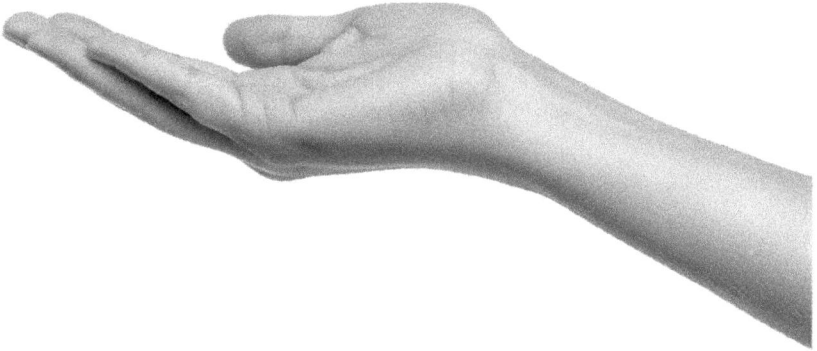

And then just **IMAGINE** that your gatekeeper, your food instinct, drifts out of your mind and lands down there on the palm of your hand.

Look at your hand.

Imagine that now.

You, the grown-up you, is looking out of your eyes at YOUR gatekeeper resting in the palm of your hand.

Maybe your gatekeeper looks like a mini you or maybe you imagine it as something else: a soldier, a security guard, a bodyguard, a bouncer.

There on your hand is the part of your mind that has been giving you all of these unnecessary and uncomfortable feelings about food.

If you could say something to this part of your mind, what would you like to say?

Have a think about that!

YOU are not giving yourself these uncomfortable food feelings … **that part in your hand is doing it**.

Write down here the things you want to say to your gatekeeper:

_____
_____
_____
_____
_____
_____
_____

To help make this process easier for you, let me share with you what many of my clients say when they imagine talking to the gatekeeper resting on their hand.

Some of them say, *'Stop it! You're driving me crazy.'*

Others say, *'I hate your guts. You've been holding me back for years.'*

Others just say, *'Let more food in!'*

STEP TWO: Talk to Your Subconscious Mind

Some people get really angry and upset. Others don't know what to say because they feel weird talking to an imaginary part of their mind.

So let me help you. If it's okay with you, I'm going to say something to that food instinct part of your mind, on your behalf.

(First question to the gatekeeper)

Firstly, I'm going to ask this part of your mind, *'**Why? Why are you doing this?** Why are you creating all of these unnecessary negative thoughts and feelings around food for this person. You're holding them back. You're giving them a hard time. They're missing out on way too much, like parties and sleepovers and school camps and going out with friends to restaurants and cafes and celebrations. They're missing out on having a good time at holidays, family dinners, work … the list goes on. **Stop it. You're driving them nuts!**'*

(The gatekeeper's response)

And this part on your hand is listening. If your gatekeeper could talk it would say, *'**Well, I'm just protecting them**. I'm just doing my best to make sure that their life is safe and predictable. I'm just keeping them away from things I think are dangerous.'*

(Second question to the gatekeeper)

*I listen to this response, and I'm confused. So I say to this part, **'But surely you must be joking?** Look for yourself. Your boss has grown up. They're mature. They don't need to* be given these uncomfortable thoughts and feelings around food anymore. **They don't need you to protect them. You're just holding them back.**'

(The gatekeeper's response)

The gatekeeper on your hand gets annoyed at my response, and says, *'**Well, you weren't there!** You weren't there when they were small and choked on food. You weren't there when they had reflux, colic and vomiting. You weren't there when the taste and texture of food made them feel nervous and anxious. You weren't there when food just felt unpredictable and unsafe. **But I WAS there!** I've been here on the inside all the time, helping and protecting. I'm just doing my job!'*

And then the gatekeeper says,

'I just try to make them feel safe. If food made them feel bad in the past, I don't let it happen again. So I keep it away. If food was around and something uncomfortable happened, I don't take any chances. I keep it away. I've got a long memory. If they get nervous or upset about anything, I keep food away. It worked when they were young, so I keep doing it. Why would I change?'

So, to you reading this book ... how OLD is your gatekeeper?

Now that you know WHY your gatekeeper is giving you these feelings around food, how old do you think it is?

Most people guess that their gatekeeper is the same age as they are now. If they are 9 now, they think their gatekeeper is 9. If they are 14 now, they think their gatekeeper is 14.

STEP TWO: Talk to Your Subconscious Mind

But this is not correct.

Your gatekeeper, the food instinct program running in your subconscious mind, is STILL the same age as when you had your FIRST negative food experience, all those years ago.

The food instinct in your subconscious mind is NOT the same age as you are today. It is much younger.

And this makes perfect sense. Because the feelings you have around food are not grown-up feelings. They are the raw feelings of that young you, when you were a baby or toddler.

The feelings you experience NOW around food are the result of decisions you made in the PAST as a baby or toddler.

So now let's bring our attention back to your gatekeeper. There it is, in the palm of your hand.

Maybe it's 3 months old or 6 months old. Or maybe it's 2 years old. We know it's young, because it's reacting to food the same way you reacted when you were young.

Maybe it was gastro or colic or reflux that made it scared of food. Or maybe ADHD and autism just made it super cautious or indifferent.

Maybe it was an uncomfortable sensory feeling you had around food and it decided to keep food away to keep you safe.

And then year after year, it continued with the same behaviour.

You grew up, but your food instinct never did.

So how do you feel about that young baby or toddler, that protective part of your mind that has never grown up? That part sitting in the palm of your hand. How do you feel about your gatekeeper?

Are you angry and upset? Or now that you understand better, do you feel a little sad? Or is it a mixture of both?

Either way, would it be okay today if we helped that part of your mind to grow up, so that it behaves like all of the other grown-up parts of your mind?

And if right now you are nodding your head and thinking, *'Yes! That's what I want!'* That young food instinct on your hand, your gatekeeper, gently says, *'Whoops, sorry.'*

It's as if this part of your mind for the first time, says, *'I'm genuinely sorry. I didn't know that what I was doing was harmful or not helpful. I was just trying my best.'*

So I wonder if I can ask you one final question?

What does this part of your mind look like? If you had to describe it or draw it, what would your gatekeeper look like?

I want you to think about that now.

Are you seeing a mini you, or are you seeing something else?

Recently I found a picture of what this part of your mind looks like. Your food instinct. Your gatekeeper.

And here it is ...

STEP TWO: Talk to Your Subconscious Mind

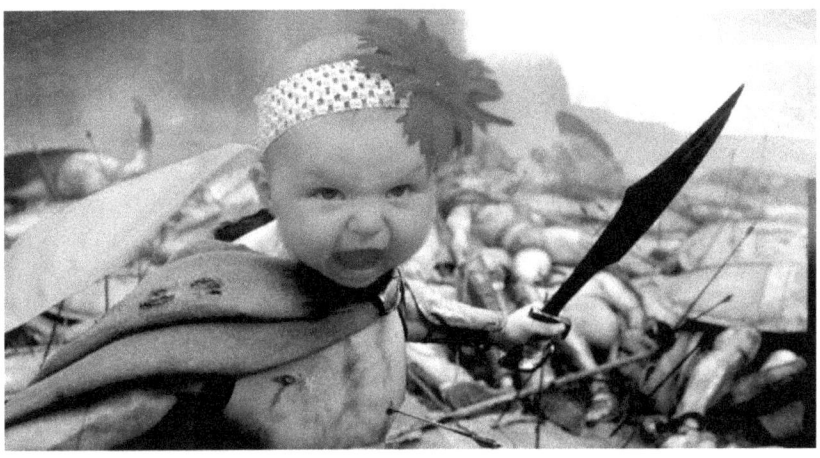

This is a picture of your gatekeeper! A young mind controlling the behaviour of a grown-up body.

If you smile as you look at this picture ... that's good!

All of these years you've been thinking that something is wrong with you, when really it's just a stubborn young part of your mind that has been doing something it believes to be right, to protect you.

It's not doing anything wrong ... it's just misdirected.

It's got the sword out. It's been protecting you from food and keeping it away for years.

But as you read through the steps in this book, your subconscious mind adjusts and finally understands.

Your gatekeeper gently puts the sword away and says, *'Whoops, sorry. I now know that I don't have to protect this grown-up you like I protected the little you all those years ago. Please forgive me.'*

But I don't want this strong part of your mind to go away. You deserve to be protected for all time by a strong instinct.

So I wonder if we can do a deal. This protective instinct can stay, as long as it agrees to just protect you from lions, tigers, sharks, crocodiles and fast moving cars, and lets you be the boss of food from now on.

Because for years, this instinct in your subconscious mind believed that IT was the boss of food.

For years, it believed that food **was as dangerous** as lions, tigers, sharks and crocodiles.

So from this moment forward, let's strike a new deal.

YOU, at the age you are right now, YOU are now the **boss of food**.

Your instinct can stay, as long as it just protects you from lions, tigers, sharks, crocodiles, fast moving cars, and anything else that you need protection from.

Your instinct has no need to protect you from food any longer.

Would that be okay?

Yes?

Good. Let's keep going.

STEP TWO: Talk to Your Subconscious Mind

Choose your future – the left or right path?

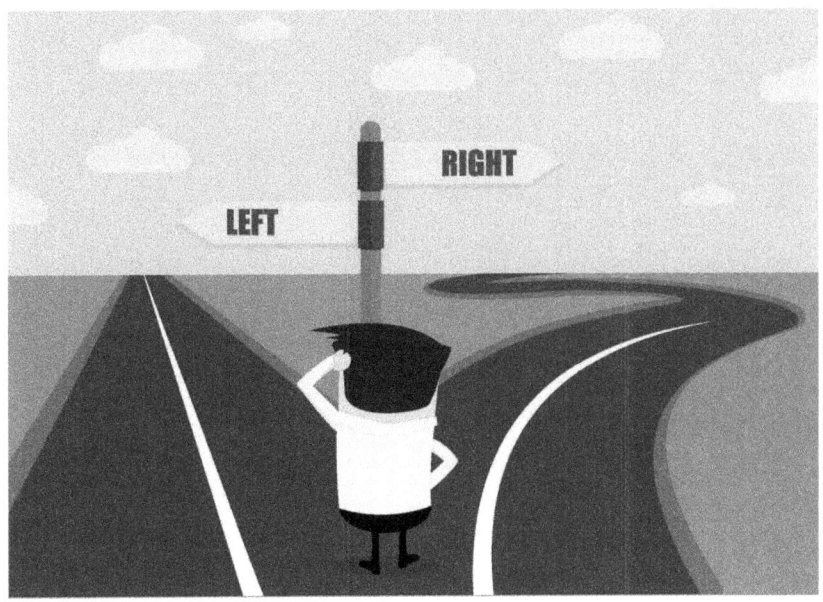

Up until now we've only been looking at the past.

You now understand that this feeling you have around food started a long time ago, in the past.

This feeling could have been created for a variety of different reasons. It may have been due to some food trauma, an overanxious nature, autism or ADHD that increased cautiousness or indifference, a heightened sensory awareness that made food feel uncomfortable. The list goes on.

But you are now in the PRESENT. And you now realise that an old, outdated 'food program' has been running the thoughts about food in your mind FOR YEARS!

You didn't know this before, but now you do.

So let's stop looking at the past, and now let's look at the FUTURE.

Let's look into your future, 10 years from now.

I want to look at two different future versions of you, 10 years older than you are right now.

Imagine you are standing at a crossroads (just like in the picture). There are two paths in front of you leading into the future. One is leading out to the left (it looks straight and appears the same as your existing path). And another is leading out to the right (it is curvy and windy and appears different to what you are used to).

The decision you make today will determine which path you take, and which future you live in.

So let's do some time travel.

I want us to speak with the two different versions of you, living two different lives 10 years into your future.

After we've spoken to both, you can make your decision.

The left path

Let's start with the left path. It's straight and looks the same as the path you've been walking for years.

Imagine you float out of your body and move down the left path. And you arrive at a time 10 years into the future.

But before we start talking to this future you on the left path, I've got to warn you about something. That future you on the

STEP TWO: Talk to Your Subconscious Mind

left path, is still being protected by that same baby/toddler feeling around food.

That young food instinct, your gatekeeper, has not changed. The same way it's been protecting you for all of your life, is the same way it keeps protecting you around food for the next 10 years on the left path.

If we could speak with that left path future you and ask, *'How's life going for you around food? Good or not so good?'*, what do you think future you would say?

Well, I think that future you would say, *'Not so good.'*

They would probably say, *'It's no better than when I was 10 years younger. In fact, it's worse. My health is not as good. My energy levels are low. It's difficult going out with friends and family to restaurants. Travelling is a nightmare. Eating at work is sometimes embarrassing. Everything that involves food in my life is difficult.'*

They would probably say they feel like a car that's got bad fuel in it. They go, but they don't go very fast. Food is like fuel. Without good food, without good fuel in their system, they're not the best version of themselves they know they can be.

I ask this future you if they have good friends in their life.

And they answer, *'Yes, but it's a problem. My friends are always inviting me to parties, celebrations and restaurants, and to go away with them on vacations. But I can't do it, because I'm always worried about food. Eating in front of people at work is also uncomfortable. I get nervous and overwhelmed. And sometimes people notice that I'm not eating and they ask me why, and I just get embarrassed. Often I just miss out. It's easier to stay at home.'*

That future you sounds like they are struggling.

If I was to ask that future you to give some advice to your young gatekeeper, to the part of your mind that's protecting you RIGHT NOW around food in that old outdated way, what would they say?

I think the future you would be firm, and say, *'Listen, I know you think you're doing the right thing. You think that the way that you're behaving and protecting us will one day magically turn around and everything will work out and we'll be happy and healthy in the future.'*

And then future you would say, *'Well, it doesn't work because I'M IN THE FUTURE AND I'M NOT HEALTHY OR HAPPY AROUND FOOD. You're over-protecting us. It's no longer helpful. Stop it. You're holding us back.'*

As you read these words and feel that they are true, something interesting starts to change in your mind.

Your subconscious mind is feeling your emotion. It's listening to your feelings.

Your food instinct, your gatekeeper is listening.

And now it understands.

It finally understands that it no longer needs to protect the grown-up you around food, the same way it had to protect the young you all those years ago. Those days are gone.

STEP TWO: Talk to Your Subconscious Mind

The right path

Now imagine that you are back at the crossroads, with the two paths in front of you. **Left** path and **right** path.

The right path is windy and curvy and looks different.

Imagine this time you float out of your body and move down the right path. And you arrive at a time 10 years into the future.

The right path is the path of the scientific eater.

A scientific eater says, *'Okay, if there's some food in front of me and I've never had it before, I'm just going to do an experiment. I might be a little bit nervous, but I'm going to use my grown-up mind to make a decision. I'm not going to let the instinct part of my mind, my past or anybody else, make that decision for me.'*

A scientific eater would say, *'If I like it, I'll eat it, and if I really don't like it, I won't eat it. It's as simple as that.'*

So let's talk to this future you on the right path. The path of the scientific eater.

If I ask this future you, *'How is life going? Is it easy or not so easy?'*, I suspect the right path future you would say that it's going pretty well.

And if I ask them what's so good about their life, they would probably say, *'Well, I've got* **freedom**. *I've got freedom to make MY decisions about life and food without those old outdated thoughts and feelings holding me back.'*

'I can go away for weekends with my friends, go to celebrations, restaurants and cafes. Work is easier, school is easier, parties are fun. I'm enjoying life. It's fantastic.'

And if I ask that future you how their body is feeling, they might say, *'You know what, when I was 10 years younger I thought I was okay. But now I've had 10 years on this right path, having more food choices, I feel fantastic! I run rings around my younger self. I feel absolutely wonderful.'*

That future you also knows and understands the body well. If there are allergies, it knows to avoid those food types. If there is autism or ADHD, it has a better understanding of the challenges without ascribing the blame entirely on food. That future you has a more realistic and mature interaction with food.

That future you on the **right path** sounds like they are enjoying life.

Making a choice

Now, in a moment, I'm going to get you to make a choice.

I'm going to get you to make an important decision.

I'd like you to decide whether you want to continue walking down the **left path** that leads to a future of no change. That leads to a future where you continue to have a difficult time around food.

OR, whether you would prefer to explore the **right path** that leads to the scientific eater you, to the path of you having freedom.

You may be nervous making this choice, so I'd like to share a true story with you that might help you get clarity.

When I'm working with an ARFID client and ask them to make a decision between the LEFT and RIGHT paths, they often

STEP TWO: Talk to Your Subconscious Mind

say, *'Why would I choose the future me on the left path? That future me is just 10 years older and their life is worse than mine. Why would I even consider choosing them? No thanks.'*

And then they say, *'**I want the future me on the right path**. That future me has freedom. They're doing all the things that I want to do. That future me is behaving as if food is like walking and breathing. It's just natural. It just happens. They don't even think about it. That's the freedom that I want.'*

BUT ... then these clients start to feel a little bit nervous and say, *'But what happens if I reach out and try a new food, and all of a sudden the old feelings come back. The nauseous feeling in my stomach. The gag reflex in my throat. The thoughts of disgust and worry in my mind. What happens if I get swamped by all of those things and I can't do it?'*

And I say to those clients, *'That's a really good question.'*

So I gently say to them, *'After everything you've heard today, you now know who it is that's been giving you all of those unnecessary thoughts and feelings around food. It's your gatekeeper, your young food instinct.'*

The client then starts to smile and nod their head and say, *'Oh yes, I get it. I understand.'*

I remind them that the way their gatekeeper protects them is by controlling their FEELINGS.

The gatekeeper knows that if it makes the stomach feel nauseous, the person won't eat the new food. That's its goal!

The gatekeeper knows that if it tightens the muscles of the throat (gag reflex) then the new food can't get in the body. That's its goal!

The gatekeeper lives in the mind. It floods the mind with nerves, anxiety, disgust and disinterest around food to keep the person away from new food. That's its goal!

> **But today, your gatekeeper has realised that you are grown-up. You are no longer that young baby or toddler from years ago. Your body has matured. Your mind has matured. You no longer need to be protected in those young, toddler ways anymore.**

And your gatekeeper today has said, *'Whoops, sorry. I've been so busy on the inside doing my job, I never looked out and saw how grown-up you are. Please forgive me. I now know I don't have to protect you from food anymore.'*

Which path do you choose?

So right now, I'm asking you to make your decision.

Imagine looking at those two paths.

Imagine looking at those two future versions of YOU.

Would you like to continue journeying down the **left path (it's easy, it's straight, nothing changes)** that leads to a lifetime of ongoing food challenges?

Or would you like to explore the **right path (it's curvy and looks different)**, the scientific eater path, that leads to the version of you that feels FREE?

Making a choice can push us out of our comfort zone.

But now you have all of the information.

STEP TWO: Talk to Your Subconscious Mind

So ...

Which do you choose?

I think I know your answer, because it's the same choice that all 2,500 of my ARFID clients have made over the years.

The choice of the right path.

And that's the path I'm helping you take your first steps on as you're reading this book.

And by reading this far, I know that you are already on your right path.

Chapter summary and key points

- ✓ Now you have a clearer picture of **your ARFID story**.

- ✓ You now understand that this feeling around food is a **'young' feeling**, not a **'grown-up' feeling**.

- ✓ You've seen a picture of **your gatekeeper**, and now it all makes sense.

- ✓ You've looked **10 years into your future** down the LEFT and the RIGHT paths.

- ✓ You are clear on what you want and have made **the right choice** for you.

Congratulations. You've completed the second step.

When we truly understand something, there is no longer any need for 'unknown' fear.

It's okay to be nervous when we do something new.

And sometimes nerves feel exactly the same as excitement.

You are now on your right path.

I think that you'll be excited about what you'll learn in Step 3.

Let's turn the page and I'll show you how to take control of your powerful subconscious mind.

Chapter 4

STEP THREE: Choose to be the Boss of Your Mind

'Expecting things to change without putting in any effort, is like waiting for a ship at the airport.'

Unknown

'The optimist sees the donut; the pessimist sees the hole.'

Oscar Wilde

This is what you will learn in Step Three

- ✓ The **power of your subconscious mind**.

- ✓ That your real power is your **power to choose**.

- ✓ You'll be surprised about what's acceptable for a **scientific eater**.

- ✓ It's perfectly **okay to be nervous** when we do something new.

- ✓ How to **take the trainer wheels off** and explore some new foods.

STEP THREE is all about stepping up and being the **LEADER**.

It's about realising that YOU are the boss of YOU.

And it's about understanding that doing something new is not about success or failure. It's about starting. It's about progress, not perfection.

Learning is a process. And you're learning to do new food.

And learning is all about just 'having a go'.

Okay, I'm here supporting you every step of the way, so let's keep going!

STEP THREE: Choose to be the Boss of Your Mind

Feel the power of your mind – the pendulum

I'd like to give you a direct experience of the power of your subconscious mind.

For this exercise we're going to use a pendulum. You can just make a simple pendulum at home. It can be a necklace with a pendant, or cotton thread with a weight on the end like a ring.

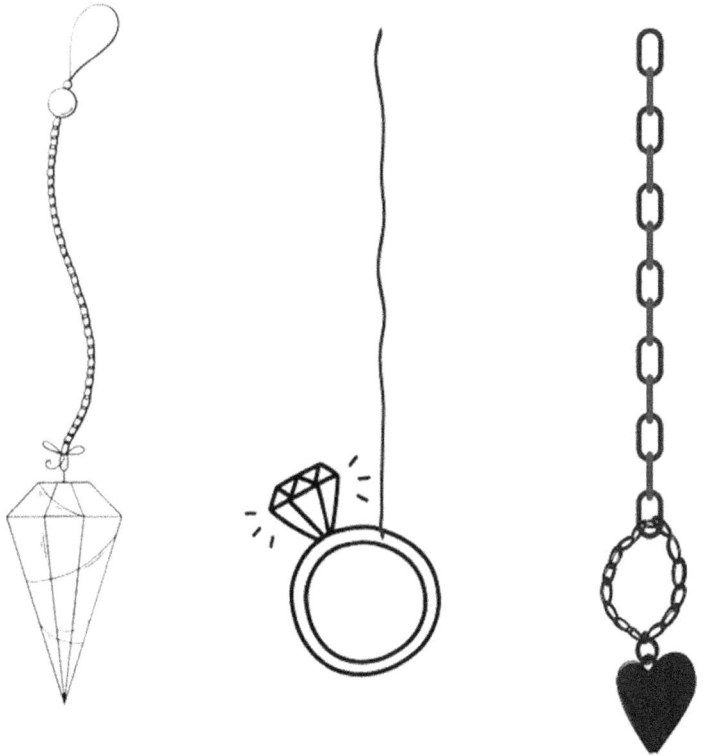

And then I'd like you to get a piece of paper, draw a circle on it with two lines. One line (a-b) going across the circle, and the other line (c-d) going up and down (see illustration).

Goodbye ARFID, Hello Food!

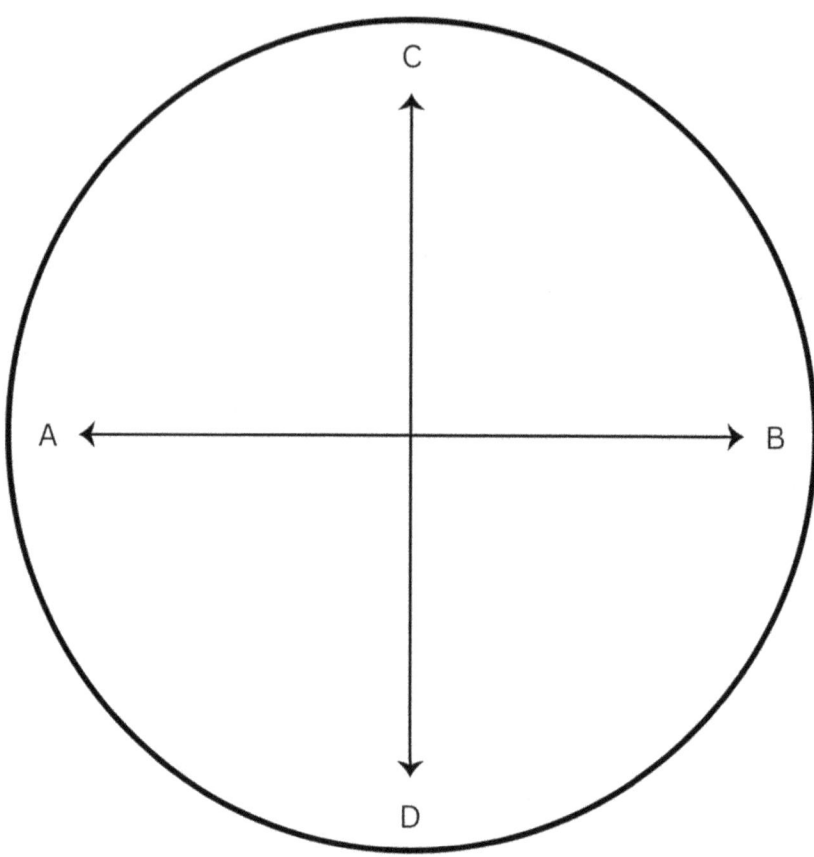

And I'd like you to hold the pendulum between the thumb and the forefinger of your dominant hand, the hand that you pick up a pen and write with (see illustration).

STEP THREE: Choose to be the Boss of Your Mind

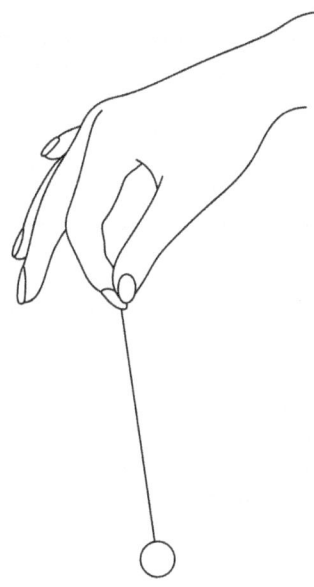

Now put the piece of paper on the table in front of you (it's more comfortable if you sit at a table while doing this exercise).

Put your elbow on the table and lower the pendulum so it touches the paper in the middle of the circle where the two lines cross.

And then I want you to focus your attention on the pendulum touching the paper.

Now slowly lift your hand up so the pendulum is about 2cm above the page.

And now I only want you to use your IMAGINATION.

Look at the pendulum and IMAGINE that it begins to swing back and forward along the A to B line.

See it in your mind. You want it to swing. You expect it to swing. Imagine it swinging … and it does.

It starts swinging. Automatically.

The more you want it to happen, the more it seems to happen, and the more you want it to happen, the easier and easier it gets. That's it.

Now, in your MIND, imagine it changing direction. SEE it in your mind going round and round in a circle. **And you're just using your mind**. And you notice the pendulum does exactly what you're thinking. Good.

Now I want you to choose a new direction. Choose diagonal or straight and imagine it swinging that way. That's right. As you focus on the new direction, the pendulum begins to change. It starts to swing exactly the way you are thinking. Good. That's it.

Now, just allow that pendulum to drop down.

If you experienced the pendulum automatically swinging, did that feel a little weird? Was that interesting?

What did that pendulum exercise show you about you and your mind?

Well, if your pendulum followed your thoughts and swung the way you were thinking, that tells me two very important things about you.

The first thing it tells me is that you have a very powerful imagination. That's going to be a benefit to you in life, and it's going to be a very big benefit to you as you follow the instructions in this book.

STEP THREE: Choose to be the Boss of Your Mind

But the second thing it tells me is way more important than that. Now I know that if you decide to focus on something and clearly set your mind on it, that you send such a strong signal to your body that your body says, *'Thank you for being so clear. Leave it to me. I'll make it happen.'*

> **Your conscious mind didn't need to know what muscles, fibres, sinews and tissues were being twitched in the arm to make the pendulum swing.**
>
> **All your conscious mind needed to do was to be very clear on what it wanted, and imagine it already happening.**
>
> **This strong conscious focus and desire helped your subconscious to influence your body to make it happen.**

So let's use your powerful mind and focus on your future. Focus on the right path.

Imagine, right now, that you are enjoying all of the good things on your right path. Maybe you're feeling good going to a party or a sleepover. Or going to a cafe or restaurant and just sitting down and feeling comfortable. Maybe you're going on vacation or a school camp, and it's easy. See yourself at a work function or going out for a wonderful dinner with somebody who's very close to you. Or maybe you're just feeling full of energy and vitality, and feeling relaxed around food.

Because when you CHOOSE to focus on the things that are important for you, and you SEE them in your mind, and you IMAGINE yourself enjoying them **right now**, you send such a strong signal that your mind says, *'Oh, really? Is that what you want? We haven't heard THAT before. Thanks for being clear. We'll go ahead and help make it happen.'*

Right now, your mind understands that the grown-up you doesn't need that nausea in the stomach anymore, so it dials it down or switches it off.

Your mind now understands that the grown-up you doesn't need the muscles in the throat contracted into a gag reflex anymore, so it relaxes them and lets them disappear.

Your mind now understands that the grown-up you doesn't need those old dangerous, disgusting and scary food thoughts, so it switches them off.

The reason I know that your mind can do this and that it is possible, is because of your experience with the pendulum.

> **Your experience with the pendulum has given you a direct experience of the power of your subconscious mind.**

Your THOUGHTS can change how your body ACTS and FEELS.

And so if your mind can do it with a pendulum, then YOU can also do it with all of the good things on your right path.

All I'm inviting you to do is to focus on the good things on your right path. Imagine they are already in your life and your mind and body will work together to make it happen.

Choice – the only thing you really own

What do you really own?

Some people would answer: my car, my house, my clothes, my bicycle, my PlayStation.

STEP THREE: Choose to be the Boss of Your Mind

But those things can all be taken away. You don't really own them.

But there is something that can never be taken away from you. And that's your power to CHOOSE.

You can choose to give up or to go on.

You can choose to be friendly or unfriendly.

You can choose to share or be selfish

You can choose to love or to hate.

You can choose to be courageous or timid.

You can choose to learn something new or you can choose to do nothing.

What are you going to choose?

If you have read this far into the book, it shows you have chosen to learn.

And by choosing to learn, it means you are open to change.

It's time to be the leader of your mind

You are the leader of your mind.

You are the boss of you.

You are now aware that you have a conscious mind and a subconscious mind.

The conscious mind is like the jockey, and the subconscious mind is the powerful thoroughbred horse.

If the jockey lets the reins loose, and doesn't give the horse any firm direction, the horse will stop or walk or gallop or go in whatever direction it wants. It will definitely not be in the race, and if it was, would have no chance of winning.

The horse needs the jockey to give it direction if it has any chance of winning the race.

The jockey is the leader of the horse. The horse is the powerful part of that combination that will get the jockey physically to the desired destination.

> **The jockey chooses the direction and the destination, not the horse.**

All the jockey has to do is to work together with the horse, to hold the reins a certain way, to sit on the horse a certain way, apply gentle pressure in a certain way. And all of a sudden, jockey and horse are off and running in the right direction, running the right race, giving themselves the opportunity to win. To succeed.

You are the leader of your mind. Your conscious mind is the leader of your subconscious mind.

There's one important quality a leader needs. If a leader doesn't have this quality, I don't think they can be a good leader.

Yes, there are qualities of respect and courage and empathy, and they're all good qualities. But if a leader is not clear on where they're going, if a leader doesn't know exactly what they want to achieve, then nobody will follow them.

STEP THREE: Choose to be the Boss of Your Mind

And so it is with you.

If you are crystal clear on all of the positive things on your right path, then this will give you (the conscious mind) a reason for reaching out and exploring food. Because if you don't have a reason for doing something, it will never happen.

But reaching out and exploring food is just the first step. It shows you that you can be a scientific eater. It shows you that reaching out and exploring food is possible.

But the **main game** is being able to do that with family and friends at dinnertime, at parties and sleepovers, at work, on school camps and in restaurants.

As you lead yourself to reach out and explore food, you find that you can begin to enjoy the main game, which is all of those important things on your right path.

What is acceptable for a scientific eater?

I'd like to help you get clear on what is an acceptable response when a scientific eater reaches out and explores new food.

😊 Like	🙂 It's OK	😐 Unsure	😒 No. Not yet
'Wow! That's good. I'll definitely have that again!'	'Not bad. I can eat that again.'	'I'm not sure I like it. I'll try it again later.'	'I don't like it. I'll try it again when my taste buds get stronger.'

The four faces in the table are the reactions that ANYBODY in the world might have when they reach out and explore a new food for the very first time.

They might try the food and say, *'Wow, I really like it!'*

They might try the food and say, *'Yeah, that's okay. I can eat that. It's not my favourite, but it's okay.'*

Or when they try it, they might say, *'Oh, I'm unsure. I probably should try it again, but at the moment I don't know whether I like that or not.'*

Or finally, they might pick up the food and when it hits their tastebuds, they know they don't like it. So they take it out and say, *'That's not for me. I don't like that. No, not yet.'*

Now that you know all about what it means to be a scientific eater, I want to ask you a trick question.

So here it is.

Which of those four responses do you think is ACCEPTABLE for a scientific eater?

1. I like it

2. It's okay

3. I'm unsure, or

4. No, not yet, I don't like it

And of course the answer is, ALL OF THEM!

There's no pressure on you to like or dislike any food you try.

Now that you understand this, you can start to use your conscious, grown-up mind, to make your decisions around food, without pressure or expectation.

You can decide whether you like it or not, rather than the old automatic responses coming up from your subconscious mind and filling you with all of the young worry thoughts that you used to have around food.

A scientific eater is really not concerned about liking or disliking. They're more interested in being curious and exploring new food.

Because when you are curious, you don't know what will happen. Nothing is predetermined or premeditated.

It's like lining up outside of a movie theatre waiting to go inside. Imagine you know nothing about the movie. You were given free tickets by a friend and you decided to take a chance and watch the movie.

While you're in the line, imagine someone comes up to you and says, '*Hey, what's the movie like?*'

You would look at them and say, '*I don't know. I haven't seen it yet!*'

When you get inside the cinema and you watch the first 15 minutes of the movie, you can start to form an opinion. Is it good? Is it not good? Are you unsure? Should you stay and watch, or is it that bad that you're going to walk out?

Now THAT sounds a little bit like a scientific eater!

As a scientific eater we don't make our mind up before we check out any food.

We just give ourselves the opportunity to explore.

Maybe we'll like it. Or maybe we won't.

One is not better than the other.

The outcomes are just a response to exploring.

Anticipatory anxiety (phobia vs. normal nerves)

In psychology there is a term called anticipatory anxiety.

What this really means is sometimes we get nervous when we do something new.

Soon YOU are going to be doing something new. As a scientific eater, you are going to be checking out foods that you've possibly never had before.

After absorbing the information in this book, your mind has begun to think differently. It's got clearer and has put a little bit of distance between you and your old food behaviours, because those behaviours are not really you. They are just old patterns of thinking that have been with you for way too long and are no longer needed.

Just by reading and thinking about the things you've learned in this book, that old feeling of anxiety that's been wrapped around this idea of food in your brain, is starting to soften and drift away. And underneath that old extreme anxiety is just normal nerves.

> **So I'd like you to remember that when you reach out and do something new, it's okay to be nervous. Because that's natural.**

And we can be nervous when we're doing something new, and we can still go and do it. But if we've got that really excessive amount of fear, then it's very difficult to push through. Just like you've been feeling around food.

This food instinct part of your subconscious mind that's been doing this old behaviour for so long, today has said, *'Whoops, sorry. I now know that I don't need to continue to protect this grown-up person like I protected them all those years ago.'*

It's time for that overprotective subconscious feeling (the gatekeeper) to soften and move away, so YOU can make conscious decisions to do something new.

And even though you might feel a little nervous, you'll notice that you'll be able to push through and do it. Or maybe you just won't be nervous at all.

Take the trainer wheels off your bicycle!

The trainer wheels on a bicycle are there to protect us from falling. But if we leave them on forever, we will always be riding the bike like a beginner.

Nobody wants to be a grown-up who is STILL riding a bicycle with trainer wheels.

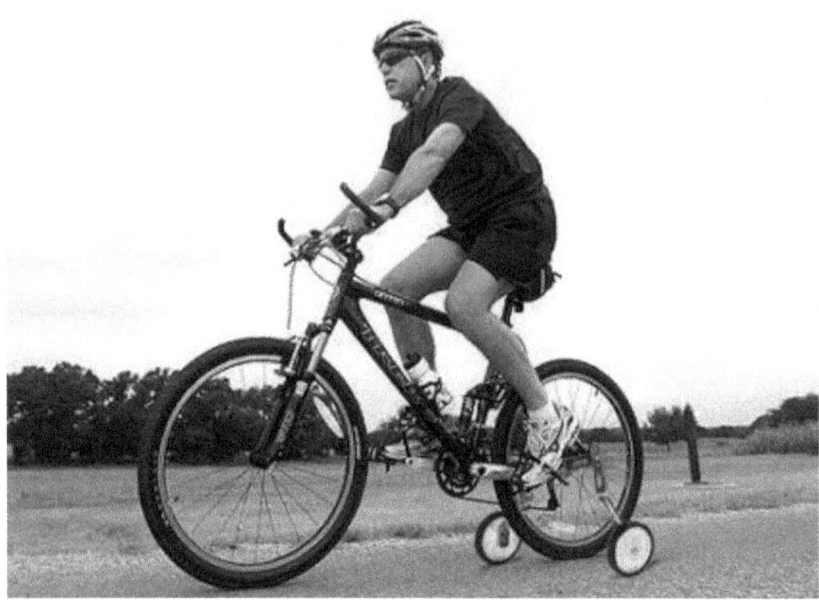

But here's the thing. When we take the trainer wheels off for the first time, something interesting happens. We get wobbly and a bit scared!

But if we persist, it starts to get easier and easier. We build confidence. We trust ourselves to keep our balance and ride.

Now that sounds a little bit like the gatekeeper and food!

When our gatekeeper finally lets go, we feel a bit wobbly and scared the first week we explore new foods. But if we stick at it, it gets easier and easier.

You now understand that you don't need your food trainer wheels (your gatekeeper) anymore. It's time to be free.

And remember: it's okay to be nervous when we do something new.

STEP THREE: Choose to be the Boss of Your Mind

Time to be a food explorer!

As you have been consciously reading this book, your subconscious has also been listening.

And if you felt some emotion while you were reading the information in this book, something interesting has begun to happen in your mind. The old automatic way of thinking has been challenged.

The subconscious mind is now taking direction from the grown-up conscious mind.

So ... time to be a FOOD EXPLORER!

I'd like you to collect about four foods that you don't currently eat and put them in front of you. You can do that now.

Start off simple. Choose foods that are like the ones you currently eat. Maybe they are a similar texture, or maybe just a different brand.

Or if you currently eat foods separated on the plate, you might want to try them together (e.g. cereal and milk, cheese on toast).

And if you're adventurous, try something new. A fruit, a muesli bar, a sandwich. Or try a food that you used to eat, but haven't eaten in a while.

And then I want you to make a copy of the Food Explorer Chart (Appendix A) so you can fill it in as you explore the new foods.

So, pick up a food, and try it now.

Let your mature grown-up mind decide if you like it or not. If you don't like it, take it out. If you like it, chew and swallow it.

And tick the column to record your experience.

Remember, ANY column is acceptable for a scientific eater. No pressure.

How was that?

You're just getting the hang of being the leader of your mind. And it's okay to be nervous. It's normal to be nervous when we do something new. But it will pass.

Try another food.

How was that? Write it on your list. Tick how you feel.

Homework

I'd like you to try one or two new foods each day for the next 7 days. If you want some ideas of foods to try, there is a list in Appendix B under 'Guidelines for trying new food'.

Most people find it best to explore new foods outside of lunch and dinnertimes. After school and at home after work seem to suit best.

This first week is about getting into the habit of being a food explorer and a scientific eater.

But if you try a food and like it … you can eat more of it!

Maybe you'll reach out and eat new food straight away. That's good. Maybe you'll be nervous and only be able to try a small amount. That's okay as well.

STEP THREE: Choose to be the Boss of Your Mind

You're in the process of learning to do something new. And you will learn in a way that matches your personality. It will be the same way you learn to do anything new in your life.

It's your race, your pace.

No judgement. Just reach out and do some exploring.

What does the recovery path look like?

The recovery path is different for every client. The process you have gone through by reading this book is designed to reduce the internal (subconscious) anxiety you have been holding towards new food.

- If your ARFID was initially caused by a physical trauma, then the information and processes outlined in this book will definitely help you begin to release the historical fear stored in your mind.

- If you have sensory processing challenges (SPD), it is normal for your current level of sensory processing awareness to be less than when you were younger. You now understand how the overwhelm of SPD may have created a hypervigilance of your young food instinct to avoid food. Hypervigilance by its nature creates anxiety. The process in this book can help reduce that 'young' outdated anxiety, so you can begin to explore foods even if you retain some sensory processing challenges.

- If you have interoceptive challenges (low hunger signals, etc.), the benefit is the same. The mature you is now aware of your interoceptive issues and can reach out for the relevant professional assistance.

With the reason for low interest in food now known, your conscious mind can begin to make different decisions. The inner mind no longer has to create additional stress and discomfort around food. Food is not the problem, it's just about managing the signals within the body. A reduction in anxiety can assist the mind/body with learning new cues.

- And if you have autism, ADHD and/or hypermobility, you can also experience the benefit from this process. Autism may create a natural predisposition to be cautious around food, but if there was additional trauma or anxiety in the past, this may have increased the natural cautiousness to an acute level. Reducing the internal (subconscious) anxiety through new knowledge and the gentle process in this book, can help you to begin exploring food again cautiously, without being held back entirely. Remember, even a small change is a step in the right direction.

So change is possible. The vast majority of my clients who go through this 3-step process experience positive change.

Positive change means that the person is able to reach out and begin to explore 'non safe' foods without being overwhelmed by their old feelings about food.

The measure of change is different depending on personality type and comorbid issues.

But with ARFID, any change is good change. And once change starts, it can be gently built upon.

The positive change from this process often helps clients get more benefit from their visits to dieticians, psychologists, occupational therapists, etc. It's as if a reduction in the internal fear opens a door for people to be able to engage better with other therapies.

But sometimes life gets in the way.

A loved one is injured, a relationship breaks down, a job is lost, a serious health crisis arises, a new choking incident occurs, you are starting at a new school … and sometimes people revert back to their old food behaviours.

It's as if the subconscious mind says, *'I've got to deal with this new crisis and make the person safe. I don't have time to put effort into doing new things around food.'* And the person slips back into old food habits, because it's comfortable and known, when things in their life are uncomfortable and not known.

Often when this client contacts me and comes in for a brief follow-up session, they are back on track quickly. It's often just a matter of getting the conscious mind back into the mode of being the leader.

Chapter summary and key points

- ✓ The pendulum has given you a direct experienced of **the power of your subconscious mind**.

- ✓ Your subconscious mind is like a thoroughbred horse, and you are the jockey. **It is time to take the reins**.

- ✓ The job of a **scientific eater** is NOT to like everything you try.

- ✓ **It's okay to be nervous when you try something new**. That's normal.

- ✓ The recovery path is different for everyone. **It's your race, your pace.** No pressure.

Congratulations. You've completed the third step.

Over the next week, I'd like you to explore some foods that you haven't eaten before. Or you can try some foods that you used to eat, but haven't eaten in a long while.

Write them on the list. Tick how you feel.

Remember, it's okay to be nervous when you do something new.

After you have explored some new foods over the next few days, go ahead and read the Bonus Section.

This will help you to consolidate all you have learned, and will help you with your motivation to keep exploring new food.

Chapter 5

BONUS SECTION:
Keeping You Strong

'When your intention is clear,
so is the way.'

Alan Cohen

'Curiosity will conquer fear,
even more than bravery will.'

James Stephens

Extra insights you'll learn in this bonus section

IMPORTANT NOTE: Only read this section if you have read all of the previous pages and have attempted to explore some new foods for at least a few days.

This next section is based on the 'follow-up' session I do with ALL of my ARFID clients.

I ask them to go home and explore one or two new foods each day for 7 to 10 days.

I ask them to record the foods they try in a food chart (example in the Appendix at the back of the book).

When they return, their two most common experiences are:

1. They have been able to reach out and explore new foods

2. They have tried some new foods but are still nervous.

The information in this follow-up session gives additional support and assistance as you explore new food.

- ✓ It will help you to **stay motivated** and on track.

- ✓ It will help **explain** the feeling you experience in the first week of trying new foods.

- ✓ It will give you **strategies** of dealing with any residual nerves around food.

- ✓ It provides parents with the **tools** needed to continue to help and support their ARFID child.

Building trust

This is what's been happening in your subconscious mind as you've been reaching out and exploring a few new foods over the past week.

Your food instinct, your gatekeeper, has been looking up at you all week thinking, *'Can I trust this person? Are they going to force me to eat things? Are they going to insist that I like everything that we try?'*

So this part of your mind is really nervous!

At the same time, YOU (the grown-up you) has been looking inwards at this young food instinct part of the mind that you've just discovered, and you've probably been thinking, *'Can I trust this little person? Are they going to stay open and let me be the leader? Will they let me decide what I want to do around food and give me the space to have my own experience? Or are they going to swamp me with all those unnecessary old feelings again?'*

Normally at the end of the first week, the two of you are beginning to work together. You're starting to TRUST each other. You're building trust.

> **And the same way that you learn to do anything in your life, is the way that you're now learning to do food.**

If you're the type of person who jumps in and just does it, then that's what you'll do with food.

But if you're cautious, perfectionistic, rigid or nervous, then that's the way you'll probably do new food.

So the first week is all about building trust. It's not about doing it fast or slow, because change is okay whether it's small or medium or large.

And of course when we learn to do something new, we've got permission to muck up and make mistakes. And that's what the first week is all about. It's about learning to do something new.

It's about not being absolutely certain. It's about being a little bit nervous but excited at the same time.

It's about exploring. And when we explore, we really don't know what to expect.

We give ourselves the **freedom to learn something new.**

Remember, it's all about progress, not perfection.

Rating food

Okay, this will be an interesting exercise for you.

I'm going to show you something about the internal part of your mind and how it thinks about food.

I'd like you to use the following table to write down up to 10 foods that you currently eat.

Think about things that you regularly have for breakfast, lunch, dinner, snacks, etc.

Done? Good.

Now I want you to go down the list and score each of these foods out of 10. One out of 10 is low (you don't like it much).

BONUS SECTION: Keeping You Strong

Ten out of 10 is the highest (you love it). But you can rate your foods with any number from 1 to 10.

Food item you currently eat	Score out of 10

Now that you've done that, I want to give you some insight into what those scores might just say about you.

If you've got none or very few, 10 out of 10 scores (which is very common for most of my ARFID clients), it shows that your mind right now lets you eat foods that are not a perfect score.

You might have foods that you scored 6, 7, 8 or 9 out of 10, and yet you can still eat them.

This is a really good sign!

It means that foods you currently eat don't need to be 10 out of 10 for you to eat them.

I'm inviting the part of your mind that lets you eat lower scoring foods to apply that same rule to new foods.

So now your mind is thinking, *'Oh, that's interesting. I already eat foods that are not perfect, that are less than 10 out of 10. So if I just take that same rule across to new foods, I can explore the new food, and I don't need it to be 10 out of 10. It's okay for it to be a 6, 7, 8 or 9, just like the foods I'm eating now.'*

Good.

However, if you notice that there are quite a few foods on your list that are 10 out of 10, then that also tells me something interesting about you.

It tells me that when you get used to a food, when you trust a food, your mind gives it a high rating. Your mind likes it, it's predictable, it's safe. But I also know that those 10 out of 10 foods on your list probably weren't always 10 out of 10.

Maybe they had to earn their spot there. Maybe you had to try them quite a few times until you got used to them, until you built up some trust.

So this might indicate that when you go and explore new foods, you need to give those new foods that same chance. Try them a few times, build up some trust, let them work their way up from a 6 or a 7 to 8 or a 9, or possibly even a 10, because it would be cruel to give them just one chance and never try them again. Sometimes, we've got to give them a few tries before we can decide whether we like them or not.

BONUS SECTION: Keeping You Strong

Plank of wood story – your 'safety net' around food

I want to tell you a story about a plank of wood. I think you're going to really like this story. It's going to start to pull all the pieces of information together that you've read and absorbed about you and ARFID.

Now that you've had a week to do some food exploring, I think you'll definitely get the (not so) hidden message in this story.

So let's imagine a plank of wood.

This plank of wood is about 45 centimetres wide (18 inches), and it's about 10 metres long (10 yards). One metre is your biggest step, so it's a pretty long plank.

And let's imagine I put this plank on the floor in my clinic. Well, it's too big for my room, so I have to open the door and this plank of wood goes out of my office and down the hallway.

And you've come to visit me in my clinic.

With the plank of wood lying flat on the floor, I invite you to stand on one end of the plank. Pretty easy, because it's 45 centimetres wide.

I then walk 10 metres down to the other end of the plank and I put a $100 note there. I look at you and say, *'If you can walk all the way down the plank keeping your feet on the wood, you can pick up the $100 and keep it.'*

So you start off and you walk down the plank easily, no problems. You pick up the $100 note and put it in your pocket. It's easy, 45 centimetres wide, no problem.

But I want to be sure, so I walk 10 metres down the OTHER end of the plank, and I put $200 down there. I turn to you and say, *'Could you just do me a favour? I just want to be doubly sure. Could you please do that again? Keep your feet on the plank, and if you walk all the way down here you can pick up $200.'*

And you think to yourself, I hope this goes on all day! This is easy money. And you walk down the plank and you pick up the $200, and you've got $300 in your pocket.

BUT I know something that you don't.

I know in the city of Melbourne there are two buildings on the west side that are both 68 storeys high. And at their closest point, they are about 9 metres apart.

So imagine I take that 10 metre plank from my office, and I go into the city, and I take it up to the rooftop and balance it between these two buildings. So it's just touching the edge of both buildings.

You and I go up in an elevator to the 68th floor. It takes a long time to go up 68 floors.

We get out onto the rooftop and look over the edge. The people down there at ground level look like ants because we're so high up.

We look at the plank balancing between these two 68-storey-high buildings. The plank is wobbling because it's breezy up there.

My colleague is on the other building and she puts a small parcel on her side of the plank where it's touching her building.

And I yell across and ask her, *'Hey, what's in that parcel?'*

And she yells back and says, *'There's $25,000 in that parcel.'*

I look at you, and I say, *'If you walk across the plank right now, 68 stories high, balancing on the top of these two buildings, the $25,000 is yours.'*

So I ask YOU a question.

If you can imagine yourself in that situation, what would you do?

Most people say, *'Well, I want the $25,000, but there is no way known I would do that.'*

And I wouldn't do it either!

The instinct in your mind would say, *'I don't care about the $25,000. I'm your instinct. I just care about your survival and keeping you safe. This is not safe. One small slip and we're dead. It's not happening!'*

So our instinct might turn our legs to jelly, make our stomach feel nauseous and sick, our head feel dizzy. It would do whatever it takes to shut down our body so we do not walk on that plank. It would fill us full of all the nervous thoughts of what might happen. And that's natural.

So, I say to you, *'Is there anything that I could do or say to get you to walk across that plank?'*

And you look at me and you probably say, *'No, I'm just not going to do it.'*

Okay. So let me give you an option.

How about if I put a **safety net** directly under the plank, and this safety net is way wider than it needs to be, the holes are way smaller than they need to be. I get it thoroughly tested by the occupational health and safety experts. They sign it off as the safest safety net in all of Melbourne. Would you do it then?

And most people say, *'Yeah, I'd give that a go.'*

And when I quiz them and ask, *'Why would you give it a go now, but you wouldn't give it a go before?'*, they would say, *'Well, it's obvious. There's a safety net. I'm not going to die. Everything's going to be okay.'*

With the safety net there, it's as if instinct takes a back step and says, *'Nothing for me to do here. It's safe, no chance of injury or death.'*

If I ask you if you would be nervous walking on the plank with the safety net underneath, you would probably say yes.

But if your instinct could talk, it would say, *'I'm not making you nervous. You're only nervous because you're doing something new for the first time.'*

Interesting.

Okay, so now we know that a safety net can make a difference to our decision making in a real-life situation.

So now I want to ask you an interesting food question.

Imagine your gatekeeper (your food instinct) drifts out of your mind and sits in the palm of your outstretched hand. Your gatekeeper is the part of your mind that USED to make you scared and nervous around food.

And I ask you, what is it that your food instinct, your gatekeeper, needs to know about the grown-up you, so that it can take a step back and say, *'Nothing for me to do here. It's safe. I don't need to jump in with the old reactions anymore.'*

> **What is the 'safety net' in your mind that would take all the fear away from you exploring new food?**

You might scratch your head and think that's an interesting question. Most people say, *'I don't really know.'*

So I'm going to give you a couple of suggestions.

Let's assume that you like plain toast.

Let's imagine you've got a piece of that toast in your hand. It's perfect. It's exactly the way that you like it. And you look at it and you think, *'I'm going to eat this toast.'*

But as it comes towards your mouth, your friend comes around the corner, doesn't see you, and bumps into you. And in slow motion the toast gets knocked out of your hand, does a double somersault, and lands on the ground and skids around in the grit and the dirt and might even land in a little puddle of mud.

My question to you is, *'Would you pick up the toast and eat it?'*

And you're likely to say to me, *'Yuck, no, I'm not going to do that.'*

And if I ask you why not, you probably say, *'It's got germs. It's got bacteria. I just wouldn't do that.'*

And I wouldn't either.

And as you're thinking and saying those things about the toast, your instinct in your mind is listening and thinking, *'That's what I want to hear. I want to know that my boss is grown-up and mature and doesn't take risks. Great, I don't need to look over their shoulder anymore.'*

So your food instinct in your mind takes half a step back.

But it wants to know a little bit more. It wants to know that it can trust you to do something else. And this is REALLY important.

So I say to you, *'Imagine you reach out and try a new food (because you are now a scientific eater). The food looks and smells okay. But when you put it in your mouth it tastes bad. It tastes disgusting. What would you do?'*

And you think about this, and you say, *'Well, I'd probably get a napkin and take it out of my mouth. And I'd probably have a sip of water to wash the taste away.'*

As you respond, your food instinct is listening on the inside and thinks, *'That's what I want to hear! I want to hear that you don't take risks, and if something tastes really bad, that you will always take it out.'*

And your instinct takes a final step back and says, *'Thank you. I don't need to look over your shoulder anymore. I can trust the grown-up you.'*

This is your safety net with new food! If you explore a new food and don't like it, take it out. Simple.

And the final thing we might share with your food instinct is this. We let it know that when you were really young, you didn't understand things like sensory processing challenges, or ADHD or autism, or hypermobility, or allergies. That young baby you didn't know any of that.

The young you didn't know that it wasn't always food's fault if you vomited, had gastro, or felt sick or nauseous.

The young you didn't know that keeping food away wasn't the best and only way to help you if you felt scared or anxious.

But the grown-up you does know all of these things.

You know and understand all of these things. So these things are not a mystery to you anymore.

They are less scary now than when you were little.

So now the grown-up you can choose to have a different reaction to things.

You know yourself so much better than that younger you, who was just reacting on instinct alone.

Manager's sandwich strategy

I want to give you a strategy. A strategy is like a plan. This is a really good strategy.

As the saying goes, forewarned is forearmed.

I want to give you a plan of how to deal with the nervous or uncomfortable thoughts that might pop into your mind, or that you might start feeling, if you reach out and try some new food.

The name of this strategy is the 'manager's sandwich'.

The reason I'm giving you this strategy is because you are now the manager of your mind.

Now a normal sandwich has got three components. It's got a bit of bread on the bottom, another bit of bread on the top, and in between these two bits of bread there's some filling. So it's got three components.

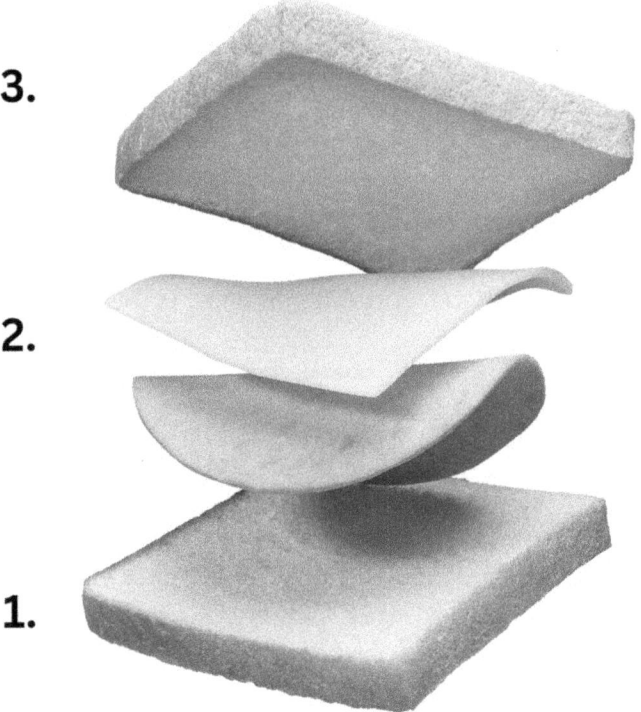

Well, a manager's sandwich has three components as well.

The FIRST part is a pat on the back.

The THIRD part is also a pat on the back.

And the SECOND part, in the middle, is a kick in the butt!

BONUS SECTION: Keeping You Strong

1.
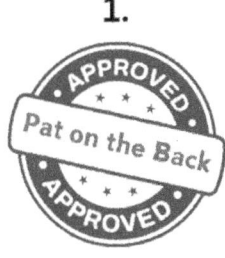

2.
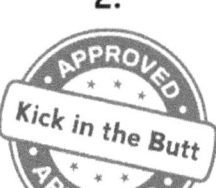

3.
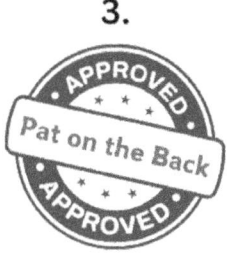

> **That's a manager's sandwich!**
>
> **A pat on the back to begin with, a pat on the back to end with, and a kick in the butt in the middle.**

I'm going to show you how to use the manager's sandwich strategy on any nerves that come into your life around food.

So let's use your imagination. I want you to imagine right now that you're reaching out and picking up a food that you've not had before. You are a scientific eater now, so this is easy for you to imagine.

But just as this new food comes towards your mouth, a twinge of those old nerves just pops into your mind. These nerves come from your gatekeeper, your young food instinct.

This is the opportunity to use the manager's sandwich strategy.

Step One – Pat on the Back

So the first thing we've got to do is we've got to pat those old nerves on the back.

And here's how we do it. We might think to ourselves, *'Hey nerves, thank you. You know what? When I was younger and there was stuff going on, I know I got nervous around food. Maybe it was a choking or vomiting episode, maybe I was just anxious, or maybe something else. It doesn't matter, but I know you got nervous of food too. You thought you had to protect me, and the way you protected me when I was small was to keep stuff away. Thank you.'*

When you say that, your food instinct probably thinks, *'Hang on. This person understands me, they love me.'*

Your gatekeeper (your food instinct) feels good about this.

Step Two – Kick in the Butt

So now we've got to kick those nerves in the butt! And here's what it sounds like.

We say to those nerves, (which come from your gatekeeper), *'Stop it! You're driving me nuts. I've grown-up now. My body has grown-up. My mind has grown-up. I don't need to be overprotected by those young thoughts anymore. They suited a young body, a young me, but they no longer help me now, because I'm grown-up. So I need you to stop it. And I need you to stop it now.'*

And your food instinct, your gatekeeper says, *'Whoa! That changed quickly. Now my boss doesn't like me at all.'* And your gatekeeper feels unloved and feels you don't understand them, and starts to get its back up.

Step Three – Pat on the Back

But we don't want our instinct to shut down, so we've got to move quickly to this next step. Here's what it sounds like.

BONUS SECTION: Keeping You Strong

We talk to our instinct and say, *'Hey, don't take that the wrong way. I don't want you to leave or go anywhere. You're super important to me. You're my instinct. But you know what? You're pretty good at protecting me from lions, tigers, sharks, crocodiles and fast-moving cars, but I'm grown-up. I do food now. I make good food decisions. If food looks dodgy, I don't eat it. If food tastes really bad, I always take it out. You can trust me. So I want you to stay and protect me from everything else, but I do food myself from now on.'*

And your instinct is listening.

Your instinct finally acknowledges that you are grown-up.

Your instinct now knows that you make good and safe decisions around food. You are the boss.

And on the inside, the two of you shake hands. You are now working as a team.

And things start to get easier and easier around food.

If you use the manager's sandwich strategy, and say it out loud with a smile and a laugh, your instinct will know that you really do understand. And those old feelings around food will just fade away.

Because you no longer need them.

Motivation ideas

1. The hokey-pokey process

This is the 'one step in', then 'one step out' process:

1. **IN**: Try it at home first
2. **OUT**: Then try it outside of home

Trying new food in a restaurant for the first time in front of family and friends might be a bit overwhelming.

So a good way to build up to the challenge is to get some takeout from the restaurant and try it at home first. And if you like it, then try the same food in the restaurant next time you go.

Your mind will think, *'Hang on, we've already tried this thing at home and everything was okay. It's safe.'*

And so you will be less nervous and you start to build confidence.

The same strategy can be used for school camps.

Get a copy of the camp foods from school, and practise eating a few of them at home in the lead up to the camp.

If you end up liking a few of the foods, it's a bonus!

It means you can eat those foods just like your friends.

It takes the pressure off and you start to build confidence.

2. Building muscle

If I go to the gym for one day and lift weights, I don't get muscles like a bodybuilding champion.

So nobody is expecting you to be the champion of eating new food after one day!

The tastebuds in your tongue are like muscles. The more you use them, the stronger they get.

Watching your muscles doesn't make them grow. We just have to turn up to the gym, do the proper exercises, and the muscles will grow in time.

Just like tastebuds. There's no need to analyse every taste from every food you try. Your job is just to explore new foods regularly and your tastebuds will mature and grow up for you.

3. Shallow end or deep end?

It's helpful to think that learning to eat new foods is just like learning to swim.

When we learn to swim, we start in the shallow end. It feels safe. The water only comes to our hips and our feet can touch the bottom.

When we learn the basics of swimming, we move to the middle of the pool. We can still touch the bottom, but the water is up to our chest. We can lift our feet off the bottom and get the feeling of floating.

Then when we're ready, we move to the deep end because we are confident with floating and swimming.

Exploring new food is just like learning to swim.

Don't jump into the deep end first. Start with foods that are similar to the ones you currently eat. Maybe start mixing them together rather than keeping them separate.

Try different brands.

Even retry foods that you may have dropped. Choose simple common foods to start with. Build up from there.

Don't put pressure on yourself to try a new food every day.

And when you find a new food you like, have it again soon. Let your mind get comfortable around the food.

Your goal is not to like EVERYTHING you try! Your goal is to get comfortable being a scientific eater. That's all.

A scientific eater can check out food without the old negative emotion getting in the way.

Have fun finding your new favourites. Each food you like is a step forward building a more confident and healthier you.

Guidance for parents

Metaphors and stories

Every ARFID child is different, so I encourage parents to connect with the parts of this book that will be helpful for their child.

This book is full of metaphors and stories. These are powerful ways to convey learning to children AND adults. Don't underestimate the emotional connection that people make to story and metaphor.

Remember that for thousands of years humans couldn't read or write. So we are hardwired to connect with meaningful stories and the metaphors they convey.

I encourage you to find a story or metaphor in this book that connects with your child, and use that as you provide daily support on the journey forward.

The concepts that children naturally connect with and find most useful are:

The gatekeeper: Most children love the picture. It gives them a fun visualisation of the part of their mind that has been making them nervous around food.

Scientific eater: A scientific eater is focused more on EXPLORING than LIKING. This change in focus takes off a lot of pressure. It can help them be curious rather than apprehensive.

Manager's sandwich: A helpful strategy that gives the child a way of speaking to the nerves that come up around new food.

The boss of food: Most children understand the 'boss' terminology. I have heard children say things like, 'Mum is the boss of me, and I am the boss of my pet dog.' When children connect with the concept that THEY can be the boss of food (rather than their gatekeeper), this gives them new empowerment.

Your child is learning something new ... mistakes will happen. The recovery path will have ups and downs.

It's important that progress is viewed in terms of following a process, rather than in terms of success or failure.

Remember, we're going for progress, not perfection.

If the child can hold the concept of being a scientific eater, then that is enough. That will open the door to EXPLORING without the undue pressure and expectation of LIKING.

For many children, when they don't like a new food, they feel they are letting themselves or their parent down. Being a scientific eater reframes this dynamic.

Any new food is okay at the beginning

When someone with ARFID decides to try some new food, any food is okay.

Some parents want to offer 'healthy' food in the beginning, but it is best to go for food that has 'meaning'.

This means food the ARFID person would see at a party or sleepover. Food they would see in the school canteen. Food from a popular takeout restaurant.

And no judgement.

Build some healthier choices in as you go along, but sweets and takeout (if they are new) is perfectly okay to begin with.

Looking at your child through different eyes

Seeing your child as a conscious mind and a subconscious mind is really helpful for parents.

Doing this can help parents see the old negative behaviour around food in a different light. They can see that the type of behaviour is out of character. It's as if the behaviour is coming from a younger person.

And it is.

Often the behaviour is what we would expect of a much younger child. The gatekeeper (in the subconscious mind) has been driving the behaviour for years.

The grown-up child, teen or adult of today is just realising this and is learning to behave and react like their current age.

Quantity, quality or just something

Don't be overconcerned with quantity at the early stage. There still may be some nerves, even when a new food is liked. Sugar and processed foods? If they are new, take it as a win.

Protect existing food

Often children think that trying new food will mean they will have to eat it in preference to their existing food.

Reassure your child that all of their existing food is safe. It will not be taken away, and will always be available for them.

Being a scientific eater just means finding some new foods that can be added to the foods they already eat.

Avoid over encouragement

Don't make the ARFID child's food exploration a centre of family attention. And don't over encourage.

Trying new foods should be just like practising a new skill that the child is interested in (e.g. soccer, Lego building, dance, etc.).

It's just something that is done regularly, and improvement comes along naturally. No forcing.

BONUS SECTION: Keeping You Strong

Chapter summary and key points

- ✓ When the subconscious and conscious minds work together, **change is possible**.

- ✓ Not all food you currently eat is rated 10 out of 10. So there is **no pressure** for any new food you try to be perfect either.

- ✓ The job of a scientific eater is **NOT to like everything** they try.

- ✓ The **manager's sandwich** is a fun and effective way to speak with the nervous food feelings in your mind.

- ✓ Your **'safety net'** is the knowledge that (1) you don't have to like every food you try, and (2) you can take food out of your mouth if you don't like it.

- ✓ You are now learning to do food again. There is no hurry. When we learn anything new, we get better and better the **more we practise.**

For the next few weeks you can continue to fill in the food explorer chart and keep track of your progress. If we do something consistently for 3 or 4 weeks, the brain creates a new 'habit'.

Now you understand that the old uncomfortable 'feeling' in your brain was just a habit that was created from when you were young. It's a habit you don't need anymore. Habits can change.

If you are already reaching out and exploring new food, you have already begun to create your new food habit. Keep going!

Cheat sheet for ARFID therapy success

Below are the key concepts and ideas you have learned in this book. By understanding and taking on board these ideas, you will set yourself up for success on your journey to say *Goodbye ARFID, Hello Food!*

No pressure

Pressure is nobody's friend on the ARFID journey.

Perception

We experience the world in our mind. Changing our mind, changes our world.

The gatekeeper (your food instinct)

Your gatekeeper is NOT the conscious you. The gatekeeper is an old protective program that lives in the subconscious mind. When you know the age of your gatekeeper, you can turn off fear and stop listening to it.

Conscious vs. subconscious

ARFID lives in the subconscious mind. When the conscious mind links new information with strong emotion, the subconscious mind can change. And change is possible at ANY age.

Scientific eater

Make your decision after the experiment, not before. And remember, any result is acceptable.

Left path vs. right path

Don't wait. Choose your future, now.

Reasons for change

Be clear on the benefits of living an ARFID-free life. This will be your motivation on the recovery path.

Trust

When your subconscious mind knows it can trust your current conscious decision-making, it will begin to release old habits.

Manager's sandwich

Be kind and firm with yourself and your inner thoughts. Your habits were created with the best intent. When it's time for an upgrade we don't blame the old computer program. We just let it go and replace it with a newer version.

Your safety net

Your 'safety net' is the knowledge that (1) you don't have to like every food you try, and (2) you can take food out of your mouth if you don't like it.

Trainer wheels

The gatekeeper is like trainer wheels on a bike. The trainer wheels serve a purpose for a short time, but are never intended to be there forever.

Nothing is wrong

You are not consciously giving yourself ARFID. It is an automatic feeling generated in the subconscious mind. The intent is positive, but the method of protection is no longer current or needed. Time to let it go.

Be the boss

The jockey leads the horse and shows it the way. And the conscious mind is the leader of the subconscious. Step up and be the boss of your mind. Be the boss of food.

Choice

Your one true superpower is your power to CHOOSE. So choose the right path. Choose what

> you want. Use the tools in this book to help you make your choice successful.
>
> **Success**
>
> It's your race, your pace. Be patient. You'll get there.

Hypnosis: uses in ARFID therapy

I am a hypnotist and I do use hypnosis in most of my ARFID therapy sessions.

Hypnosis is a powerful way for information to be accepted directly by the subconscious mind without the conscious mind filtering and intruding.

Hypnotherapy is the combination of hypnosis and therapy. Taking someone into a relaxed hypnotic experience can provide a portal for releasing unwanted past emotions and behaviours, which can then create an opportunity for absorbing new information to take life in a new and more positive direction.

I take all of my ARFID clients through the 3-step process and tailor each session to their specific ARFID type and comorbid presenting issues. Towards the end of each session I take the client into hypnosis to give the subconscious mind the maximum opportunity of absorbing all the learnings and information of the session. Letting go of the past, and 'seeing' the future done differently.

However, I have a confession to make.

The 3-step process you have learned in this book is usually sufficient by itself to help most of my ARFID clients experience positive change, without the need for hypnosis.

For most of my clients, the positive mental shift of releasing old ARFID thoughts and behaviours has already occurred BEFORE the hypnosis part of the therapy commences.

How is this possible?

It's because the stories, metaphors, insights, education and emotion generated by the 3-step process are enough by themselves to help most people to begin to release their old ARFID behaviours.

Many of my younger clients (aged 7 to 10) keep their eyes open during the hypnosis component. And yet they still experience positive change from the therapy session.

Hypnosis is a wonderful tool for consolidating all of the learnings and insights contained in the 3-step process.

And for many clients, the experience of being in hypnosis convinces them of the power of their subconscious mind, and so strengthens their resolve and the outcome.

This book is enough by itself to help you let go of your old ARFID behaviours. However combining the 3-step process with hypnosis is a powerful way to help the mind be free of old behaviours, and enjoy life as a true scientific eater.

If you want to experience the hypnosis component of the 3-step process, you can choose one of the following 3 options:

1. Download the ARFID therapy hypnosis audio recording, so you can immerse yourself in the hypnotic experience at home
2. Obtain access to the full video course of ARFID Food Phobia Therapy (which contains the hypnosis audio)
3. Book in for your personal ARFID Food Phobia Therapy session with Glenn Robertson and experience ARFID hypnosis tailored individually for your specific circumstances.

Details of all three options can be found at the back of the book.

Afterword

You've reached the end! Well done.

For many people, just reading this book will give them a new understanding about ARFID, and will open the door for change.

If that's your experience, great. Keep going!

Go back and read the parts of the book that resonate with you the most. Use the strategies to help you with any challenges on your new food journey.

If you need more support, you can reach out and join the ARFID Australia Support Group on Facebook where I am the administrator (details in the following pages).

And if you want to explore and experience in more depth the different ARFID therapy options I have available, keep reading and I'll give you the details.

Warm regards,
Glenn

Acknowledgements

In no particular order, I'd like to thank and acknowledge a number of people who have travelled with me on this ARFID journey of discovery.

To the many thousands of ARFID clients I have worked with I extend my heartfelt thanks. You continue to be a source of inspiration and learning. The ARFID therapy I provide has evolved over the years in response to the diversity of ARFID challenges presented by each and every client I see.

The reason I am working in the ARFID area is because of a chance meeting with Felix Economakis (Registered Psychologist based in London, UK) in 2017. I saw Felix present his ARFID process at a hypnosis seminar in Melbourne, Australia. I was impressed that his process worked just as effectively with or without hypnosis.

Felix has been an inspiration and friend for many years. The core steps of his ARFID process are the inspiration for the 3-step therapy process outlined in this book.

Dr Rob McNeilly is well known in the Ericksonian hypnotherapy field as an author, trainer, teacher and provider of professional industry supervision. I am grateful to Rob for sharing his insight and guidance with me over the years. Rob's focus on keeping the complex simple and empowering the client to change through curiosity and positive expectation, is a style I aspire to with all of my clients.

The work of Dr John Sarno has also been an inspiration to me in shining a light on how the subconscious mind can make decisions independently of the logical, conscious mind in its endeavour to help and protect the individual.

Hanlie, my wife, is also a professional therapist and is a constant positive influence in all of my undertakings. She patiently listens to my daily therapy musings and has provided important editing and feedback as this book evolved. Thank you Hanlie.

And finally to Margaret, my mother. Mum was the epitome of moral strength and love, and was an active supporter of my work in the ARFID field for many years. Her legacy and gift of unconditional support is the mindset I take into every therapy session. Thank you Mum.

About The Author

Glenn is married and enjoys being in a blended family of 4 children and (so far) 3 grandchildren.

For the past 15 years Glenn has been the principal therapist at Specialist Hypnotherapy helping people make rapid changes to their negative behaviours, habits and emotions.

The ARFID therapy 3-step process has been used by Glenn with over 2,500 ARFID clients internationally and within Australia.

Glenn's educational ARFID videos have over 300,000 views and he is the administrator of Australia's largest ARFID Support Group with over 6,000 members and families.

Currently Glenn is Australia's leading ARFID therapy provider combining hypnosis with psychology phobia release protocols.

Glenn conducts personal ARFID therapy sessions in his clinic in Melbourne, Australia, and remotely via Zoom. He also provides recorded video and audio ARFID therapy options through ARFIDtherapy.com

And finally, Glenn is an amateur apiarist, a beekeeper. He enjoys the intricacies and mysteries of the 'hive mind' and sharing organic honey with family and friends.

Glenn's websites:

ARFIDtherapy.com

SpecialistHypnotherapy.com.au

Email: glenn@ARFIDtherapy.com

Glenn as a Speaker

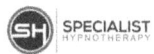 **SPECIALIST** HYPNOTHERAPY

GLENN ROBERTSON

Australia's leading ARFID Specialist combining hypnosis with phobia release therapy

www.ARFIDtherapy.com

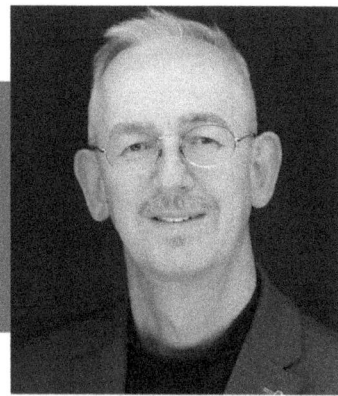

EXPERIENCE

Glenn has worked with over 2,500 ARFID children (aged 8+), teenagers and adults within Australia and internationally. Most of Glenn's ARFID (Avoidant Restrictive Food Intake Disorder) clients experience a reduction in their lifelong food anxiety within one or two therapy sessions.

STORY & PERCEPTION

Altering a person's perception and giving them a new internal story around their unwanted behaviors & emotions, creates an opportunity and expectancy for change by:

- giving a new understanding of the roles of the conscious and subconscious minds
- introducing the person to their powerful 'instinct'
- showing clients how to speak to their subconscious mind
- increasing options by giving back the power of choice

LET GO OF THE PAST

Glenn uses the same simple 3-Step Process to help clients **overcome other eating challenges** (bulimia-BN, binge eating disorder-BED, food/sugar addiction, overeating/overweight), **let go of past trauma** (bullying, relationship breakups, personal loss, parent/sibling conflict), and **overcome phobias** (insects, animals, driving, flying, needles, public speaking, etc).

HEARING GLENN SPEAK

Glenn shares the simple 3-Step Process that helps his clients to release their unwanted limiting emotions and behaviors, and be free to start living life differently.

His stories are an inspiration to anyone who thinks that change is not possible. Listening to Glenn speak provides the inspiration that by altering our perception, change is possible for anyone at any age.

PRESENTATIONS

HEALTHCARE
Glenn's presentation is relevant for Healthcare workers who want to expand their thinking on helping clients.

SCHOOLS
Glenn's presentation is entertaining and relevant for secondary school children to learn about the power of their mind.

BUSINESS
Glenn gives a new perspective to adults on the reasons for their unwanted emotions and behaviors by dispelling the victim mentality and empowering them to choose change.

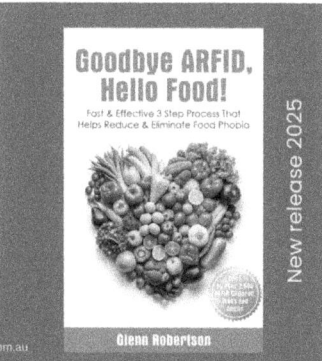

SpecialistHypnotherapy.com.au   Glenn@SpecialistHypnotherapy.com.au

ARFID Therapy, Products, Resources and Assistance

If you feel the need to reach out for more information and support with ARFID, the following pages contain resources and therapy information to assist you moving forward:

1. Special offer: free ARFID roadmap

2. Free video: What is ARFID?

3. Personal: 2-session ARFID Food Phobia Therapy program with Glenn Robertson

4. Support group membership: ARFID Australia

5. Audio book: *Goodbye ARFID, Hello Food!*

6. Audio recording: Hypnosis ARFID

7. Full online video: ARFID therapy

Special offer – free ARFID roadmap

The free ARFID roadmap booklet gives you an informative and visual understanding of ARFID, and explains how you can **let the ARFID feelings go quickly**.

You can download your FREE copy of the 26-page ARFID roadmap booklet from ARFIDtherapy.com

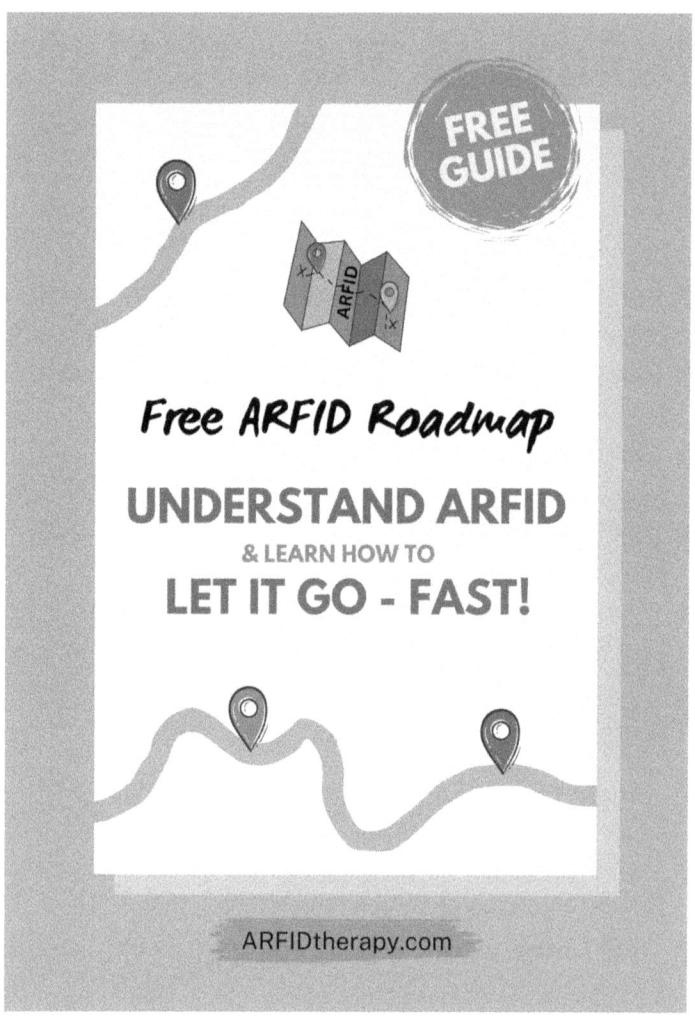

Free video – What is ARFID?

In 2019 I created a short animated ARFID information video called 'What is ARFID?' and posted it on YouTube.

The video is 13 minutes long. At the time I created the video I was told by marketing advisers that nobody would watch a 13-minute video, and that I should shorten it to 2 minutes.

They said that if I posted a 13-minute video, I might get 500 views at most.

However, I argued that people with ARFID would watch the video because it was educational and provided hope and support for those seeking answers and therapy options.

Well … at last count the video has over 250,000 views and is **the most watched ARFID video on YouTube**.

Go to ARFIDtherapy.com to get your direct link to the 'What is ARFID?' video.

After reading this book, I think you will find the video helpful and insightful.

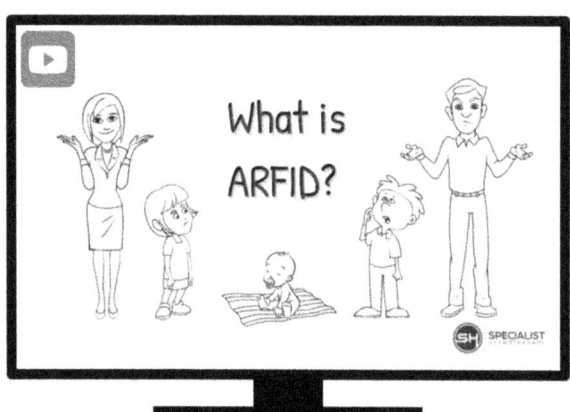

ARFID Food Phobia Therapy with Glenn Robertson

Experience live, the 2-session ARFID Food Phobia Therapy program that combines hypnosis with psychology phobia release protocols.

The program is personalised to your ARFID type and takes into account any comorbid issues that may have contributed towards the development of your ARFID.

The program includes:

- Individual 2-session ARFID Food Phobia Therapy program personally delivered by Glenn Robertson

- Insight and understanding into how your mind works to help you let go of ARFID

- Specialised ARFID audio take-home recording

- Hypnosis (where appropriate) forms part of the initial session

- Email Q&A access for 30 days after therapy

- Membership of the ARFID Australia Support Group

- The goal of the therapy is for you to experience more comfort in exploring 'non safe' foods after just one or two therapy sessions

- The therapy is appropriate for children 8+ years of age, teenagers and adults

ARFID Therapy, Products, Resources and Assistance

- Efficacy and success of the therapy is consistent whether provided in clinic or via Zoom

- Join over 2,500 ARFID clients who have already participated in this positive therapy experience.

The program can be completed in-person in the Melbourne clinic with Glenn, or it can be undertaken remotely via Zoom, Australia-wide and internationally.

Go directly to ARFIDtherapy.com to obtain more information and access the online appointment booking link, or scan the QR code below.

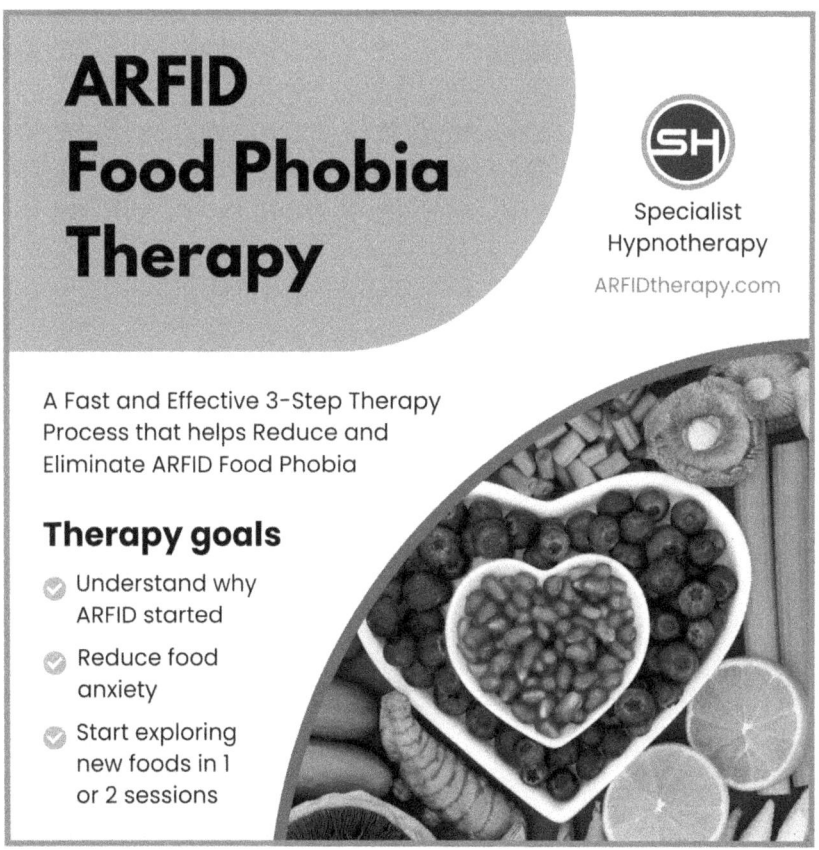

Goodbye ARFID, Hello Food!

ARFIDtherapy.com

Complimentary 15-minute Zoom discovery call appointment

All potential clients can connect for a complimentary 15-minute Zoom discovery call to ask questions before booking the session, and to determine if the therapy is appropriate for them or their child.

ARFID Australia support group

If you're looking for a supportive and helpful group to be your 'sounding board' as you start or continue your ARFID recovery journey … you've found it!

This group is for adults with ARFID and the carers and parents of children/adolescents with ARFID.

Although the title of the group says Australia, members from all countries will gain benefit from the resources and connections they find here.

With over 6,000 ARFID individuals and families, the ARFID Australia support group is a private and secure place to connect and learn.

Your purchase of the *Goodbye ARFID Hello Food!* book will give you automatic membership into the group.

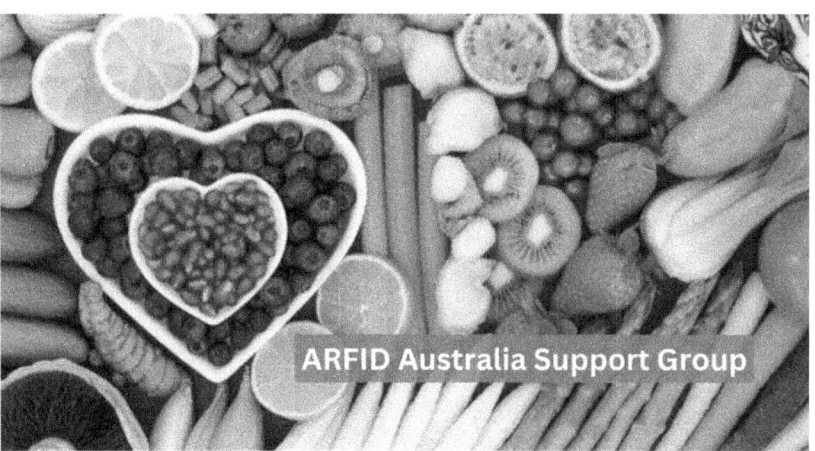

Goodbye ARFID, Hello Food!

ARFID Australia Support Group

ARFID therapy online options

If you prefer ARFID therapy and support in the comfort of your own home, then some of the below options may be suitable for you.

a. Audiobook: *Goodbye ARFID, Hello Food!*

If you prefer to listen to books rather than read them, then the audio recording of *Goodbye ARFID, Hello Food!* is for you.

Glenn's voice brings the book to life and gives you a more personal connection to the stories, metaphors and information contained in the book.

ARFIDtherapy.com

b. ARFID hypnosis audio recording

If you want the hypnosis experience of the ARFID therapy 3-step process, this is a perfect accompaniment to this book.

After reading the book, you can immerse yourself in a hypnotic experience as you listen to Glenn's voice connecting with your subconscious mind and reinforcing all the positive stories and metaphors contained in the 3-step process.

This is not the audio recording of the book. It is a separate recording of the same ARFID therapy hypnosis that clients experience in their personal ARFID therapy session with Glenn.

It is beneficial to listen to this recording once per day for 7 days to help the key concepts of the ARFID therapy to lock into the subconscious mind.

ARFIDtherapy.com

c. Full video recording of the ARFID Food Phobia Therapy program

If you want a recorded version of the full ARFID Food Phobia Therapy program, then you can access a full video recording of the entire 2-session program, including all bonus material.

You receive lifetime access to all content for less than the cost of the live 2-session program with Glenn.

This is beneficial for children who can rewatch parts of the therapy to understand key concepts they may miss on just one viewing, or one session.

Watch as many times as you need, and use the bonus material to keep you motivated on your new food journey.

ARFID Therapy, Products, Resources and Assistance

There are two versions of the hypnosis audio recording provided in this program, one for primary aged children, and another for teenagers and adults.

Scan the QR code to go to ARFIDtherapy.com and connect with the private membership site where you can start watching the ARFID Food Phobia Therapy 2-session program immediately in the comfort of your home.

ARFIDtherapy.com

Appendix A

Food Exploring Chart

Date	Number	Food name	😊 Like	🙂 It's OK	😐 Unsure	😟 No. Not yet
			'Wow! That's good. I'll definitely have that again!'	'Not bad. I can eat that again.'	'I'm not sure I like it. I'll try it again later.'	'I don't like it. I'll try it again when my taste buds get stronger.'
	1					
	2					
	3					
	4					
	5					
	6					
	7					
	8					
	9					
	10					
	11					
	12					
	13					
	14					
	15					
	16					
	17					
	18					
	19					
	20					
	21					
	22					
	23					
	24					

Appendix B

Guidelines for trying new foods

The best way to approach trying new foods is to have the mindset of a 'scientific eater'. A scientific eater does an experiment (tries the food) and THEN makes up their mind.

It's best to start with just trying one or two new foods each day. But if you feel comfortable, you can try more.

And remember, there is no pressure to LIKE the foods. Nobody likes every food they try. The goal is to calmly try the food (like a scientific eater) and then decide if we like it, if it's just okay, if we are unsure, or if we don't like it. Sometimes we might have to take a few bites to see if we actually like it. That's okay. That's normal.

And it's normal to be a little bit nervous the first time we try something new. That's okay. But there is a big difference between feeling a little nervous, and feeling full of fear. After the ARFID therapy you still may feel nervous sometimes (that's normal), but you will find that the fear that has prevented you from trying foods in the past has diminished or disappeared.

As you keep trying one or two new foods each day, you will begin to build up a few foods that you like. You can then start to gradually eat these foods a bit more regularly.

And remember ... not all food has to be new. It is okay for the food you try to be a variation of something you already eat, like the bread you currently eat but with a different filling, or instead of the plain pasta you may like, you can add a little sauce to it and check it out.

It's also okay to explore food you used to eat, but have dropped. This is also a great way to start exploring foods again.

Here are some food ideas to get you started.

Sandwiches

Try different types of bread, white, wholemeal, etc.

Sandwiches can have a simple spread like vegemite, jam, honey, peanut butter, etc.

Or the sandwiches can have cold cuts of meat like ham, roast beef, roast chicken, etc.

The sandwich can also have salad (by itself) or with cold cuts. The salad can consist of any of the following: lettuce (iceberg is easiest), cucumber, tomato, grated carrot, etc.

Sandwiches can also be toasted, like cheese, ham & cheese, etc.

Fruits

Watermelon, mango, pineapple, oranges, kiwi, strawberries, apples and mandarins are statistically the fruits that most people like to start with, and have the highest success rate.

Hot foods

If the family is cooking and eating curries (chicken, beef, vegetarian, etc.) then a portion of these can be kept and tried. The same goes for foods like stir fry, spaghetti bolognaise, lasagne, etc.

Home-made pizzas are also a good option. You can buy the bases from the supermarket. Oven bake the base first to make semi crispy, then add toppings of your choice and heat. Spread on some tomato paste and add mozzarella cheese, ham and pineapple for a Hawaiian pizza. Or try combinations including salami, capsicum, mushroom, etc.

Burgers (homemade) or from a takeaway are also a good food to try. Start with just the burger and bun and systematically add cheese, lettuce, tomato sauce, etc. as you get more adventurous.

Dairy

Yoghurts (especially probiotic yoghurts) have a high success rate. Always buy full cream yoghurt rather than the low or no fat varieties (full cream yoghurts taste much better).

Crackers with cheese are a good option to try.

Different sorts of flavoured milk are also nice to try – strawberry, chocolate, etc.

Vegetables

Steamed or cooked vegetables are better than raw. Vegetables can be tried by themselves, or with salt/pepper, or an appropriate sauce (cheese sauce, etc.). Vegetables can also be tried in a soup.

Roast potato, roast or steamed pumpkin and green beans are a good place to start.

Individual salad vegetables can be tried, but it is more common to eat salad vegetables in conjunction with others. Greek salad is good to start with, although the feta and olives may initially be a strong taste for some. A garden salad is nice and simple (lettuce, tomatoes, cucumber, grated carrot). All salads will benefit from a small sprinkle of dressing. French dressing is mild and easy to start with. Balsamic is also popular.

Nuts

Peanuts, walnuts, cashews, almonds, etc. are an easy snack and good to try. You can try them raw, roasted or salted.

Muesli bars

Muesli bars (health bars) are convenient and good for snacks. There are many different varieties of flavours and ingredients.

Eggs

Eggs can be tried scrambled, fried or poached. Sometimes it is nice to have them on toast. Eggs also benefit from a sprinkling of salt.

Pastry goods

Sausage rolls, pasties, meat pies are also good foods to try.

Testimonials

'Wow!! I saw Glenn Robertson today for the first time and cannot believe the results! Life-changing!

I was sceptical before going, so many times in the past I've got my hopes up and things haven't worked out. I've added more safe foods over the last couple of years but for 26 years I pretty much lived on bread and butter.

With Glenn today I had to take 7 foods that I would normally not go near. I managed to try all 7 without gagging.

After the session I went to McDonald's and had a cheeseburger for the first time ever!!

Thank you so much Glenn, life-changing!

I recommend to anyone who has AFRID to go and see Glenn. Miracle worker! I still have a long way to go and my tastebuds will take a while to get used to everything but already so excited with the results I'm seeing.'

Luke Y – Sydney, Australia

'I just wanted to give Glenn Robertson a huge thank you for his time and patience with me during my session with him back in October.

Glenn you have completely changed the way I view food and have helped me become closer to family and friends.

Since I have seen Glenn, I have felt so much more comfortable trying foods and have even picked up some new favourites. I'm expanding my selection and able to travel more to see my family knowing I'll always be able to find myself food. It has been truly some of the best couple months of my life.

So thank you so much Glenn. And thank you so much to everyone in the ARFID Australia Support Group for the support and encouragement. I'm so grateful to have found this group and finally have been able to get a session with Glenn.'

Bella P – Gold Coast, Australia

'We had the ARFID therapy appointment, all very relaxed and worded in a way that children understand.

My daughter (9) was nervous going in but by the end was very relaxed and happy. Every question was asked after seeking permission, so the child was very much in control.

I am still in shock. The way she threw the piece of apple into her mouth, chewed and swallowed it with no anxiety made me and hubby look at each other with a look of WTF!! And then her casually asking to try a McChicken with no lettuce made me think what magic was cast?!

The main thing was her doing it all with a smile on her face and no signs of fear or anxiety.

Testimonials

Thank you, she was amazing and we are so proud of her. Glenn did it all in such a way that there is no pressure but gives her the confidence to try.'

Emma N – Christchurch, New Zealand

'My son (14) had his first session with Glenn today and it was amazing!

He spoke to my son with the utmost respect in a calm and caring manner. He checked in on him every step of the way and made sure my son was comfortable the entire session. He has such an extensive knowledge of ARFID.

At the end of the session my son tried 3 new foods and 1 new drink he hasn't been able to have in a long time. I had to hold back the tears as I could not believe what was happening right in front of me.

The way my son just reached for the foods with no hesitation was something of a miracle on its own. He has even tried something new for dinner, and ate half of it.

If you are considering whether to take this path or not, I would highly recommend it if you can. I would do it again in a heartbeat.

THANK YOU Glenn!'

Leonie L – Melbourne, Australia

'Just posting because I've had the most amazing 36 hours of my life.

My son and I saw Glenn Robertson yesterday. My son is 11 and was restricted to pretty much vegemite on toast, hot chips and sweet biscuits.

It had been lifelong and was the biggest stress in his and my life.

As well as ARFID, my son also has a diagnosis of ADHD, ASD, hypermobility and low tone.

This session was life-changing. So amazingly life-changing, I can't even explain it in words.

He has tried 5 foods since his session – that he wanted to try! Even the mention of trying anything previously would have been met with a full-blown panic attack, rocking back and forth in the foetal position and it wouldn't have happened. I have been working with allied health for years and his diet has got more restrictive not less. No amount of bribes helped – he would rather have starved.

It's been so hard. Five foods is just incredibly unbelievable.

He had hot chips for lunch and said, 'What does sauce taste like?' And tried the sauce! He didn't like it – but we just reassured him that was okay and that his tastebuds were still learning about new foods.

My son has never tried sauce in his life. Usually he can't even sit near sauce and would have a panic attack if it was on him or touching him, let alone try and eat some!

We have never in his 11 years had a family meal together. His 8-year-old sister burst into tears today when he said he wanted to try a hot chocolate.

Glenn you have made such a massive positive impact on our family. I cannot even explain it. Thank you, thank you, thank you.

If you are even considering seeing Glenn for your child please do it. It is worth a shot.

If my son could even be more comfortable sitting near foods we would have been ecstatic. His fear was that crippling.

I burst into tears at the end of the session and had to leave the room many times over the last day to cry – so many happy tears.

How this will affect and change his and our family's lives is just immeasurable. I cannot wait to see what the future holds. Even if this is as good as it gets, it's already so much better.

That happiness I see in his eyes is someone who has so much less fear in his life. His life has been transformed.'

Tegan D – Tasmania, Australia

'I just wanted to thank you so much for the therapy session.

My whole lifestyle has changed already and I've been feeling so much more confident and happy with my relationship to food.

My social life and relationships have already improved as I don't feel anxious to eat in front of people anymore, as well as being able to eat some of my previously most feared foods!

I can't thank you enough for your expertise and guidance on ARFID.'

Esther T – Melbourne, Australia

'My 17-year-old boy has had severe restricted eating since he was about 2 years old. His safe foods were limited to Up&Go, Jatz, milk, Weetbix, Nutella on Milk Arrowroot biscuits, ice cream, an occasional apple (which has only been the last year or so), and home-baked cookies. We also managed to get him to eat one brand/one flavour of puréed vegetables, again it was occasionally.

He was diagnosed with autism at the beginning of last year, after 6 months of OT and a session with Glenn Robertson he is eating scrambled eggs that he cooked himself and a selection of fruit and veggies (he also will eat apple, blueberries and apricots).

He told me he is so proud of himself and I can't tell you how proud I am!'

Kylie P – NSW, Australia

'It's been a week yesterday since we first went to see Glenn Robertson at Specialist Hypnotherapy and I'm completely blown away.

We have seen such a huge shift in my boy's (10) mind and a massive reduction in anxiety around trying new foods.

Testimonials

This kid who has been on less than 10 foods and drinks for much of his life is sticking new foods into his mouth, chewing and swallowing!

If he ever tried anything previously it was a reluctant nibble, usually followed by a spit. But now he is taking big bites! I am literally laughing as I write this as it is such a change it is almost unbelievable. He even tried sushi of all things!

He hasn't liked everything he's tried and there's still a way to go in incorporating those foods he likes into his everyday diet but wow this is the biggest step forward we have ever seen in him. He even took an apple to school for fruit time and ate it! He hasn't eaten a fruit in 5 years!'

Kate C – Tasmania, Australia

'I want to thank you publicly for literally changing my life.

Your passion to help people who suffer from ARFID is truly a gift. You have taught me how to see the world differently, in doing so I now treat me differently.

The most important gift you gave me was peace of mind, and I will be eternally grateful.'

Karen C – NSW, Australia

'My daughter (8) had her first session with Glenn this afternoon.

I was absolutely blown away at the end of the session to watch her eat half a hot cross bun, a small bowl of Sultana Bran with milk and a few bites of a muesli bar. I was speechless and cried tears of joy, especially when she asked if we could go out for dinner for which we did and she ordered spaghetti.

I feel fortunate in that we had about a dozen safe foods before our session (lots more than others I know). Prior to this her diet only consisted of white and yellow foods but now her future looks brighter!

I am beyond thankful to Glenn Robertson and highly recommend him to anyone considering going down this path. Now to keep exploring!'

Sarah R – QLD, Australia

'I have just been to a session for my 16-year-old ARFID daughter with Glenn Robertson at Specialist Hypnotherapy and feel like I have witnessed a miracle!

One 2-hour session and she sat up to a table of fear foods and proceeded to eat them without hesitation or anxiety. Curious about the food's smell and taste!!

Thank you so much Glenn for releasing my girl from the confining ARFID rules. I hope it continues and am incredibly grateful for the opportunities you have opened up to her now.'

Christine N – Victoria, Australia

'Today we saw Glenn Robertson for hypnosis ARFID therapy.

It was a huge day for my 12-year-old son who has ARFID and has only eaten 3 foods since he was 18 months old.

He tried 7 new foods after the session, he sat there calmly and without gagging. He didn't like them all but are on the list to keep trying.

He keeps telling me that it's really weird how that wall that stops me from trying food is not there anymore, and that his tongue and tastebuds will get used to different flavours in time.

He is so excited to be starting this new journey and knows that it's something that can get better and will get better and he now knows that he is in control.

So if anyone is struggling with food I say please give this a go. Thank you Glenn, you are a wonderful caring man and my son really was engaged with you throughout the session.

It's a long road but we are on the right path to success.'

Jane M – Victoria, Australia

'Just wanted to give some feedback on our recent experience with Glenn Robertson at Specialist Hypnotherapy.

My 20-year-old son suffers with ARFID and has since the age of 4. Although I have taken him to see doctors, child psychologist, dieticians etc., we were still at a standstill as to what to do next.

After constant research of our own, I came across Specialist Hypnotherapy and life for my son right now couldn't be greater. One single virtual session with Glenn, has changed his life. He has made some incredible changes over the past few weeks, changes that we never thought we would ever see!!

My son's safe food was KFC and a few other unhealthy sad choices. He always struggled with the smell of other people's food, or the look of what they were eating. He was always anxious about food and wanted to eat good food but just could not do it.

Over the past two weeks, since his session with Glenn Robertson my son is now eating steak, cucumber, salad, crumbed fish fillet, ribs, fried egg, healthier cereals, he is even mixing food on a plate which he would never do. He is still incorporating a few of his safe foods and choosing something different off the KFC menu with the goal to eventually have it every now and again.

Even that fact that he now uses a knife and fork to cut up and eat his food makes me so excited!

My son is now talking about joining the gym and has a less anxious but positive outlook of his future health. It has been such an emotional beautiful experience.

We are so very grateful for Glenn Robertson's amazing work with our son. He truly made my son feel okay about his situation and helped him get through this. He is happier and less anxious. He actually asks me, 'What's for dinner Mum?'

Thank you Glenn Robertson and Specialist Hypnotherapy for your amazing work with our son. We would highly recommend your services to anyone who is in this situation.'

Roseanne S – NSW, Australia

'Anyone who is thinking about booking a session with Glenn Robertson I cannot recommend him more highly.

My son (9.5, ARFID, ASD, ADHD) had a 2-hour Zoom session with Glenn 6 weeks ago, followed by a 45-minute session a week later.

The therapy session went really, really well.

Glenn is so calm and gentle and tells a lot of stories. The therapy went for 2 hours. I wasn't sure if Zoom would work for my son but he paid attention the whole session.

I was very cynical about whether my 9.5 year old would try new foods at the end but he did calmly try 6 new foods, including a bite of cheese pizza which was a big win.

In the days and weeks following his sessions with Glenn my son has initiated trying new foods. He is up to trying about 35 new foods (some easier, some harder than others). He has been able to do things like eat cheese tacos at a family gathering (it's been over a year since he last ate cheese).

My son also goes to sleep listening to a recording from Glenn for ARFID kids, and I think this is helping consolidate what he learnt during the sessions with Glenn.

To anyone thinking about booking a session with Glenn – do it!!! I think my son is a good age for it.

I wondered if I would've been better off flying to Melbourne for an in-person session but my son engaged really well over Zoom so I think I agree with Glenn that Zoom can be just as effective as face-to-face.'

Sarah P – NSW, Australia

'I would like to share something phenomenal and life-changing that happened to our son yesterday.

After struggling for over a decade with "fussy eating" our son was finally diagnosed with ARFID earlier this year.

Over the years we have spent hundreds and hundreds of dollars on "eating specialists", CBT, food exposure treatments, you name it we have done it.

In the end, I found Glenn Robertson from Specialist Hypnotherapy.

We were prepared to fly our son to Melbourne for the therapy with Glenn, when I discovered he was offering treatment to ARFID sufferers in Perth.

After a couple of months wait my son finally had his therapy with Glenn in Northbridge yesterday.

I sat with my son during his therapy and watched as the miracle unfolded, with him trying more than 4 different foods by the end of the session and honestly looking like a new boy!

His tiredness seemed to lift away, he was filled with hope and excitement about the future. I cried then and I cried with joy all the way home as I told him more times than I can remember, how proud of him his dad and I were.

This will change our son's life. His energy levels, his brain power, his school life, behaviour, his social experiences like camps and birthday parties, holidays without a separate suitcase full of "safe foods", maybe ditch the vitamin and mineral supplements and hopefully he will now be able to sit with us at the dinner table with our (once) "smelly foods".

A new journey has just begun and my mummy cup has been refilled to the brim. So very, very proud of our boy! So happy!

Thank you Glenn from the bottom of my heart.'

Julie B – WA, Australia

Notes

Goodbye ARFID, Hello Food!

Notes

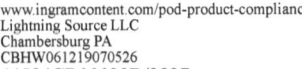